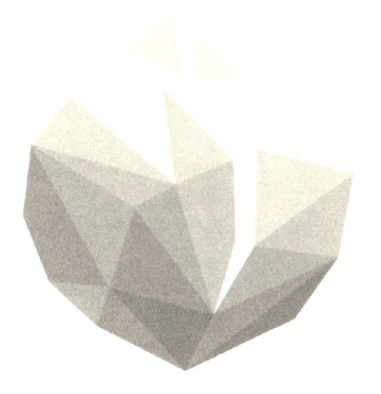

The Badass Body Goals Journal: Booty Shaping & Resistance Training

Created with love by
Jennifer Cohen, Amir Atighehchi, Ari Banayan, & Mikey Ahdoot

Copyright ©2019 Every Damn Day, LLC

All rights reserved.

Published by Every Damn Day, LLC.

No part of this publication may be reproduced, or stored in a retrieval system, or transmitted in any form or by any means, electronic, mechanical, recording, photocopying, scanning or otherwise, without express written permission of the publisher.

For information about permission to reproduce elections from this book, email team@habitnest.com

Visit our website at www.HabitNest.com

PUBLISHER'S DISCLAIMER

While the publisher and author have used their best efforts in preparing this book, they make no representations or warranties with respect to the accuracy or completeness of the contents of this book. The advice and strategies contained herein may not be suitable for your situation. You should consult with a professional where appropriate. Neither the publisher nor the author shall be liable for any loss of profit or any other commercial damages, including but not limited to special, incidental, consequential, or other damages.

The company, product, and service names used in this book are for identification purposes only. All trademarks and registered trademarks are the property of their respective owners.

SPECIAL THANKS

We'd like to extend a wholehearted, sincere thank you to the entire Habit Nest team for all their help in creating this journal. We love ya!

ISBN: 9781950045990

THIRD EDITION

Exercises Disclaimer:

The exercises provided by Habit Nest™ & Jennifer Cohen (and habitnest.com) are meant to serve as a general guide and are not to be interpreted as a recommendation for a specific treatment plan, product, or course of action. Exercise is not without its risks, and this or any other exercise program may result in injury. They include but are not limited to: risk of injury, aggravation of a pre-existing condition, or adverse effect of over-exertion such as muscle strain, abnormal blood pressure, fainting, disorders of heartbeat, and very rare instances of heart attack. To reduce the risk of injury, before beginning this or any exercise program, please consult a healthcare provider for appropriate exercise prescription and safety precautions. The exercise instruction and advice presented are in no way intended as a substitute for medical consultation. Habit Nest™ disclaims any liability from and in connection with this program. As with any exercise program, if at any point during your workout you begin to feel faint, dizzy, or have physical discomfort, you should stop immediately and consult a physician.

While this is an exercise guide, it is not intended to be a direct fit for each person. It is imperative that each person tweaks the program to work for them in a way that suits their personal needs best, especially from a safety standpoint. Do not perform any exercises that cause you pain in any way. Consult with a certified personal trainer to help guide you through each exercise in person to assure they are all being done properly and in ways that will minimize injury.

Information Disclaimer:

The information provided by Habit Nest™ (and habitnest.com) is for educational and entertainment purposes only, and is not to be interpreted as a recommendation for a specific treatment plan. Habit Nest™ does not provide specific medical advice and is not engaged in providing medical services. Habit Nest ™ does not replace consultation with a qualified health or medical professional who sees you in person, for the health and medical needs of yourself or a loved one. In addition, while Habit Nest ™ frequently updates contents, information regarding health and fitness changes rapidly, and therefore, some information may be out-of-date. Please see a physician or health professional immediately if you suspect you may be ill or injured.

The Habit Nest Mission

We are a team of people **obsessed with taking ACTION** and **learning new things** as quickly as possible.

We love finding the **fastest, most effective ways** to build a new skill, then **systemizing that process for others**.

With building new habits, we empathize with others every step of the way *because we go through the same process ourselves*. We live and breathe everything in our company.

We use our hard-earned intuition to outline **beautifully designed, intuitive products** to help people live **happier, more fulfilled lives.**

Everything we create comes with a mix of **bite-sized information, strategy, and accountability**. This hands you a simple yet **drastically effective roadmap** to build **any skill** or habit with.

We take this a step further by diving into **published scientific studies**, the opinions of subject-matter **experts**, and the **feedback we get from customers** to further enhance all the products we create.

Ultimately, Habit Nest is a **practical, action-oriented startup** aimed at helping others take back decisional authority over every action they take. We're here to help people live **wholesome, rewarding lives** at the **brink of their potential!**

– Amir Atighehchi, Ari Banayan, & Mikey Ahdoot
Cofounders of Habit Nest

Table of Contents

1   *The Key Factors of Fitness Success*
- *The Unvarnished Truth*
- *Which Booty Shape Do YOU Have?*
- *A Little Booty-ology*
- *How We're Going to Get You the Best Butt Ever*
    - *Top Reasons People Have Trouble Shaping Their Butts*
    - *Testing for a Glute Imbalance*
    - *Important Steps for Getting Your Glute Muscles Firing*
    - *Angling*
- *Building a Strong Core*
- *How Often Should I Exercise?*
- *How the Journal Works*
- *Sample 4-3-2-1 Workout*
- *Resistance Training*
- *At Home Workouts: Alternative Exercises for Resistance Training Days*
- *The Two Primary Factors That Determine Your Progress*

21   *Optimizing Every Aspect of Your Nutrition*
- *Some Basic Fat Loss Science*
- *Macronutrient Ratios*
- *Taking Action on Your Nutrition Goals*
- *Effectively Tracking Your Progress*
- *Adjusting Based on Your Progress*

39   *Getting Started*
- *Goal-Setting Principles*
- *Perfectionists, Tread Lightly*
- *Holding Yourself Accountable*
- *Developing Strength from the Inside Out*
- *You Are Perfect as You Are*
- *The Three Factors of Behavior Change*
- *General Safety Tips*
- *The Extreme Importance of Form*
- *Commit*

53 The Workouts
- *Workouts 1 - 10 + Check-In & Pro-Tip*
- *Workouts 11 - 20 + Check-In & Bonus Challenge*
- *Workouts 21 - 30 + Check-In & Pro-Tip*
- *Workouts 31 - 40 + Check-In & Bonus Challenge*
- *Workouts 41 - 50 + Finished!*

163 Fin
- *So... What Now?*
- *Meet the Habit Nest Team*
- *Shop Jennifer Cohen / Habit Nest Products*
- *Share the Love*

170 Workout Index
- *Glute Activation Warmups*
- *4-3-2-1 Exercises*
- *Resistance Training Exercises*
- *Stretches*

Our Mission In Creating This Journal

Sometimes, it isn't easy to get to the gym.

Sometimes you're not sure what to do when you work out.

Sometimes when you exercise, you don't feel like pushing yourself.

Our goal in creating this journal was to make it as easy as possible for you to have an amazing workout every day, watch incredibly fast progress happen right before your eyes, and ultimately feel supremely confident in your body.

We created this all in one personal trainer & tracker so that you don't have do ANY thinking when it comes to your workouts.

Having the journal removes any possible excuse for having an awesome workout, because the journal itself provide people a way to keep competitive with yourself so you can continue to see progress without plateauing.

There is no guess-work. Your ONLY mission is to just find the time to open the book and do a 25 minute workout. If you can make the commitment to create the time, open the book, and start the first exercise, you'll find yourself pushing harder than ever before without even realizing how it happened.

We created this journal to help you actually achieve your ultimate fitness goals.

The Key Factors of Fitness Success

The Unvarnished Truth

Whether you have a naturally athletic build, a figure that's curvaceous, or one that's willowy, there's good news:

You can develop most of the physical attributes you've always wanted but didn't get from Mother Nature or your gene pool.

The truth is, with strategic work, anyone can become fitter, stronger, more toned, more self-assured, and sexier.

That's an outcome that's realistic and healthy — for anybody.

With the right physical and psychological moves, you can turn the body you have into the body you want - losing inches, dropping pounds, and developing a stronger, more sculpted look and greater mental fortitude in the process.

If the goal of getting fit, shaping your lower body, and trimming your waist has seemed too daunting in the past, you were probably going about achieving it in the wrong way.

Sorry to lay that on you, but it's *the unvarnished truth*.

Maximizing your fitness potential isn't as difficult or taxing as many people make it out to be.

It involves four critical elements:

1. A blend of strength-training workout,
2. The right type of cardiovascular exercise,
3. Targeting your muscles at different angles to achieve the exact look you want, and
4. Consistency.

Combine these cornerstones of fitness with healthy eating habits - upgrading the nutritional quality of your food choices by using food primarily as fuel, eating regularly, snacking strategically, and you'll soon be on your way to a leaner, stronger, fitter physique with a chiseled waist line and tight tush.

Which Booty Shape Do YOU Have?

The reality is that we each come in different, beautiful shapes and sizes. Our booties look different based on our skeletal structure and the amount of muscle and fat on our differing bodies. But no matter the shape of your skeleton, you can change the way your butt looks through diet and the right type of exercise.

Think of it like this - someone who is 4'11" obviously has different possibilities for the way their body can look than someone who is 5'11". But, both of these people still have the potential to transform their bodies in ways that maximize their potential.

The Four Main Shapes of the Derrière:

Although you should be able to pick out which type of booty you have from these pictures, even if there isn't an *exact* match, these are only meant as a guide. We're all too different to have exact categories we each fit into!

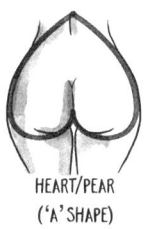

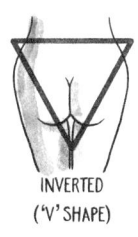

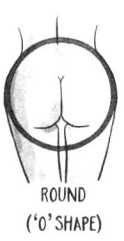

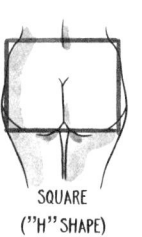

HEART/PEAR	INVERTED	ROUND	SQUARE
('A' SHAPE)	('V' SHAPE)	('O' SHAPE)	("H" SHAPE)

The Heart/Pear 'A' Shape: This type of butt results from fat distribution around the lower portion of the butt and thighs, leading to an increase in widening from the waist down to the bottom of the butt. Underdeveloped heart/pear shaped butts are commonly referred to as 'Saddlebags'.

The Inverted 'V' Shape: The 'V' shape becomes more common as we age because lower estrogen levels change the place of fat storage from the butt to the midsection. It gives the look of the bottom of the butt being less full than the top, resulting in a 'V' shape.

The Round 'O' Shape: Also known as 'the bubble butt', this type of booty is the result of fat distribution around the whole butt cheek.

The Square 'H' Shape: This shape is the result of prominent hip bones (the structure of the pelvis) and distribution of fat in the hips (also known as love handles), giving the more vertical look on the sides of the glutes.

No matter which type of booty you do have, we're going to make sure to get you the booty shape you *want* to have.

A Little Booty-ology

Let's take just a moment to talk about about your derrière.

It's really important to understand a little bit about how vital butt health is to the functioning of your body, and get familiar with the different parts of the booty that need to be developed for the best overall shape and size.

Your butt is made of pure muscle, and is probably the most important muscle in your entire body.

But your booty isn't just one muscle - it's a combination of three primary muscles groups called:

The Gluteus Maximus: The biggest muscle in the area, responsible for extending the leg backwards and rotating the pelvis and thighs.

The Gluteus Medius: Located on top of the gluteus maximus that raises the leg out and to the side, while promoting overall body-balance.

The Gluteus Minimus: Residing under the upper part of the gluteus maximus, it works with the gluteus medius.

Although the Gluteus Maximus is the largest muscle in the area, all three muscle groups are important to both your every day functioning, and the shape of your butt.

Strong glutes help support the core, decrease your risk of serious injury, improve posture, and of course, help your butt look great in any outfit.

Regardless of your genetics, you can shape your butt any way you want if you understand the different shapes your booty can take and create a plan of action that will steer you towards your goal.

In the next section, we'll discuss why so many people struggle with getting results and help you understand exactly how we're going to get you the look you want.

How We're Going to Get You the Best Butt Ever

The TOP Reasons People Have Trouble Lifting, Shaping, and Toning Their Butts

There are many reasons you may not be seeing optimal results thus far:

1. Not 'activating' the glute muscles (not firing the glute muscles)
2. Muscle imbalances
3. Training methods that don't work
4. Repeating the same movements over and over again
5. Not enough resistance training
6. Over-training the gluteus maximus and under training the gluteus medius, gluteus minimis, hamstrings, and adductor muscles
7. Not eating well enough
8. Not training consistently enough
9. Incorrect technique and form, causing compensation with the other muscle groups such as the quadriceps

Failing to activate your glute muscles causes other muscle groups to overcompensate, which is the absolute easiest way to delay your progress and potentially injure yourself, too.

The second biggest problem leading to a lack of results is not targeting each part of the glute muscles with a variety of exercises to hit the butt muscles at every possible angle.

Testing for a Glute Imbalance

Glute imbalances lead to a failure to activate the glute muscles.

Glute imbalances are very common because of the simple fact that our sedentary lifestyles cause our butts to become 'dormant' over time.

Consistently sitting for long periods of time causes the hip flexors to tighten and the glute muscles to weaken, leading to decreased strength and stabilization in our butts.

Some Words Like 'Butt'

- Rear End
- Hind End
- Hiney
- Glutes
- Posterior
- Rear
- Can
- Cheeks
- Derrière
- Fanny
- Bum
- Butt
- Behind
- Ass
- Arse

This decreased strength and activation of the glute muscles leads to muscle imbalances and an assortment of injuries to our lower back and legs.

Here are some exercises to determine whether you have a glute imbalance, or difficulty activating or firing your glute muscles:

1. Stand on one foot with one leg lifted for one minute. Then do the same thing with the other leg.

2. Get into a table-top position with your hands directly underneath your shoulders. From here, pull your abs in towards your spine so your back is straight, and extend one leg up while contracting the glute muscles in that leg as tightly as possible. Then, perform the same movement with the other leg.

3. Air Squats: Standing up, separate your feet so that they're shoulder-width apart. Keeping your back straight and your toes pointed straight forward, bend your knees so that your butt goes down towards the floor. As you perform the movement, make sure your knees are moving straight up and down rather than bending forward past your toes. Complete the movement repeatedly until it burns too much to do anymore. When it gets difficult, pay attention to whether you lean to one side of your body as you complete the movement.

<u>After performing these exercises, answer the following questions:</u>

1. In the first exercise, was there one leg you felt more stable on at the end of the minute?

2. When completing the exercises above, do you feel contraction in your glute muscles or does it feel like your hamstrings and/or quadriceps are doing all of the work?

3. When performing the first two exercises, did you have an easier time contracting one side as compared to the other?

4. Do you feel that your glute muscles on one side are bigger or stronger than the other side?

5. When performing the air squat exercise, did you favor one side of your body over the other by leaning in that direction?

If your answer to any of the above questions is 'yes', chances are you have some level of a glute imbalance and/or difficulty activating your glute muscles. Without correcting glute imbalances and making sure you're *activating* the glute muscles, your legs and booty cannot transform into the shape you want because the right muscles aren't being properly trained. Imbalanced or uneven glutes won't just affect the quality of your results, but they'll impact ability to properly and safely perform pretty much any lower body exercise! Our program combats the issues that arise from glute imbalances by specifically taking steps to ensure your glutes are 'activating' properly as you perform each exercise.

Now, let's talk about 'Glute Activation'

The harsh reality is that most people don't actually activate the muscles in their butts when doing their workout routine.

When someone really understands the importance of glute activation, it adds a whole new quality to their tushy workouts.

Glute activation is just a fancy phrase to represent the idea that the muscles in your butt should be working or 'firing' properly when you perform exercises intended to target those muscles.

Activating the glute muscles is like waking them up from a deep sleep so that they're ready for the workout. It's just like drinking coffee in the morning, except for your butt!

Important Steps for Getting Your Glute Muscles Firing:

1. Building the mind-muscle connection

When you want to do any physical movement, your brain releases a neurotransmitter called **acetylcholine** that stimulates the muscles to move.

What's remarkable is that research has found that the more active attention you place on the muscle you want to move, the more acetylcholine the brain releases.

In other words, the more mental attention you give to your butt muscles as you're performing each repetition of an exercise, the better the muscle contracts and 'fires.'

So, bringing your mind into your booty as you workout is crucial!

2. Loosening up your tight butt muscles and making sure they're firing

You loosen your butt muscles and activate them by completing simple movements that allow you to really *feel* the glute muscles contracting so you can aim to feel the same contraction throughout each exercise.

We're going to begin each workout with a **resistance-band warmup** to wake your booty up so your entire lower body is primed for the best possible results.

The good news: Because the glutes are the biggest muscle in your body, they have the most room for change. The results will come quickly if you put in the work!

Angling

One of the problems many people have with training their butts stems from thinking of their butt as one muscle.

In reality, the butt is made up of a group of different muscles that each require unique movements from every direction to target the different parts for the overall best possible shape.

You need to make sure to target and develop each muscle that makes up your butt.

*By incorporating unique variations of each exercise,
we'll make sure that you're targeting each key part of the butt and leg muscles consistently so that your entire lower body is being developed for the best possible results.*

Building a Strong Core

If you really want to develop a strong core - which is an essential part of almost every physical movement you make throughout the course of your day - you need to challenge all the muscles in the abdomen.

- *The rectus abdominis* (the two bands of muscle that run down the center of your abdomen),
- *The transverse abdominis* (the muscle that wraps horizontally around your lower abdomen), and
- *The internal and external obliques* (which form the innermost and outermost layers that run down the sides of your waist).
- *The Mid & Lower Back*

In other words, to build true core strength you need to work the muscles that are deep inside your core, not just the superficial muscles.

Building a strong core is important for lots of reasons.

For starters, the muscles in your core (your whole torso) provide the girdle or corset that supports your entire body.

Developing a powerful core can reduce your risk of experiencing lower back pain or other injury.

By contrast, neglecting these crucial muscles can shortchange you of the stability your body needs for a variety of movements in daily life.

Having a weak core is like turning off your body's power center and trying to rely only on satellite forms of energy instead (by compensating for physical movement with other muscles that the core should be the primary factor in).

Keep in mind though, that if ripped abs are your goal, no amount of core training guarantees you'll get them.

Abs aren't necessarily 'made' in the kitchen - the muscles themselves are developed in the gym. BUT, without working just as hard in the kitchen as you do in the gym, your abs won't ever show the way you want them to!

How Often Should I Exercise?

This is a common question that is situational based on what's realistic for each person.

The journal is structured to be undated and used by what works for you, your goals, and your schedule.

As a frame of reference:

- **Light**: Exercise 2 days a week.

- **Medium**: Exercise 4 days a week.

- **Hard**: Exercise 5-6 days a week.

If you're driven enough to achieve the best results, you should set a long-term goal of building up to 5-6 workouts a week.

How the Journal Works

Every day, you're going to be given a complete workout routine consisting of:

1. How long the workout will take
2. Exactly which exercises to perform
3. Images showing how to perform each exercise
4. The duration of each exercise
5. The optimal duration for your resting periods

You have two tasks to complete on days you choose to workout:

1. <u>Before you get to the gym (or right before you start)</u>:
   Look at what the day's workout consists of - which exercises you'll be doing - and read the explanations in the workout index in the back of the journal. Alternatively, you can visit the 'Exercise Guide' link listed on each page which contain video walkthroughs of how to complete each exercise for that day.

Until you're familiar with each exercise, it'll be annoying to keep looking back at the index during your workout so it would be wise to get familiar with the exercises the night before or for 5 minutes before you begin.

2. <u>During your workout</u>: Fill in the amount of repetitions you did for each exercise. You could either do this quickly after each exercise, after each set, or during the 30s break following each circuit.

We designate tracking lines for all of this, you just have to write down the numbers. This is one of the ways you'll be tracking your progress to see how far along you've come!

You can see the flow of a sample workout on the next page.

Sample 4-3-2-1 Workout

Three of the *five* workouts for the week will be what we call the '4-3-2-1' method. *Each of the workouts will have a warmup followed by four circuits, broken down as followed:*

Begin 3-5min Warmup

GLUTE ACTIVATION WARMUP (30s EACH)

1a. Clam Opener

1b. Glute Bridge w/ Band Flutter

1c. Tabletop w/ Donkey Kick

1d. Lateral Leg Raise

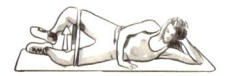

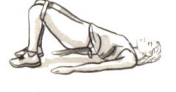

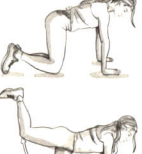

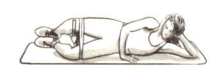

(30s Each Side)

(30s Each Side)

- 30s Each Leg (w/ Foot Flexed)
- 30s Each Leg (w/ Toes Pointing Down)

Begin '4-3-2-1' Workout

<u>Circuit 1:</u> Perform these four exercises for 60 seconds each.
(*You'll do this entire circuit **once** with no break in between exercises*).

CIRCUIT 1 (60s EACH)

1a. High Knee

1b. Bulgarian Lunge

1c. Bulgarian Lunge

1d. Side V-Up

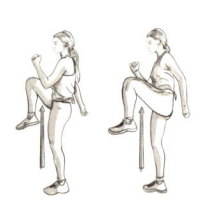

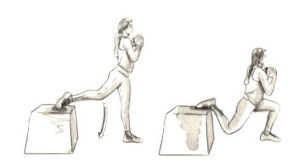

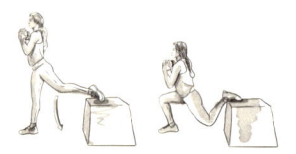

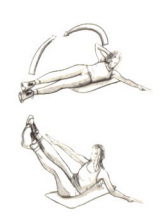

REPS: _____ → REPS: _____ → REPS: _____ → REPS: _____
                (Right Leg)   (Left Leg)   (30s Each Side)

Now, take your first break for 30 seconds.

Circuit 2: Perform these three exercises for 50 seconds each.
*(You'll do this entire circuit **twice** with no break in between any exercises or sets).*

CIRCUIT 2

2a. Side Shuffle w/ Floor Tap

2b. Plank Step Up

2c. In and Out Jack

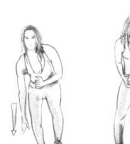

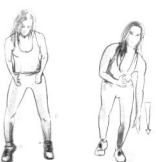

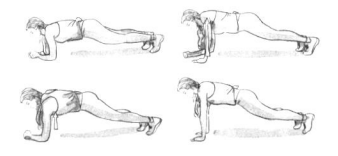

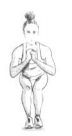

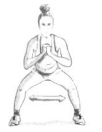

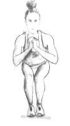

SET 1 REPS: _____ → SET 1 REPS: _____ → SET 1 REPS: _____

SET 2 REPS: _____ → SET 2 REPS: _____ → SET 2 REPS: _____

Now, take your second break for 30 seconds.

Circuit 3: Perform these two exercises for 40 seconds each.
*(You'll do this circuit **three times** with no break in between any exercises or sets).*

CIRCUIT 3

3a. Side Plank w/ Torso Twist

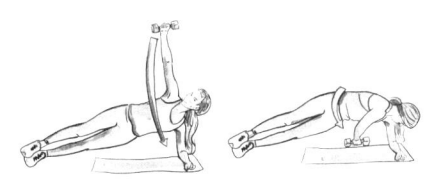

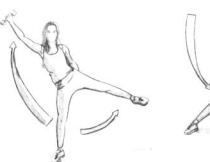

3b. Lateral Lunge w/ Half 'X'

(Left Side) SET 1 REPS: _____ → (Left Side) SET 1 REPS: _____

(Right Side) SET 2 REPS: _____ → (Right Side) SET 2 REPS: _____

(Alternate Side) SET 3 REPS: _____ → (Alternate Side) SET 3 REPS: _____

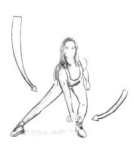

Now, take your third break for 30 seconds.

Circuit 4: Perform this one exercise for 30 seconds.
(*You'll do this circuit **four times** with a **15 second break** in between each set*).

CIRCUIT 4

4a. Pendulum Jack

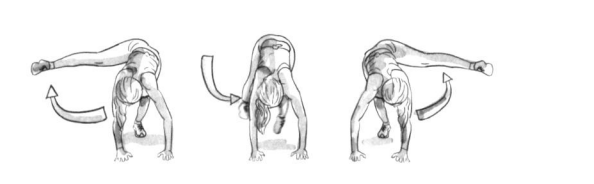

SET 1 REPS: _____ → 15s REST
SET 2 REPS: _____ → 15s REST
SET 3 REPS: _____ → 15s REST
SET 4 REPS: _____ → 15s REST

Now, take your fourth break for 30 seconds.

Begin Cool Down

COOL DOWN

1a. Hamstring Stretch   **1b. Runner's Stretch**   **1c. Butterfly Stretch**   **1d. Lat Stretch**

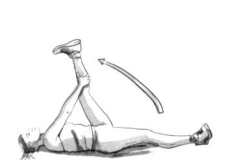

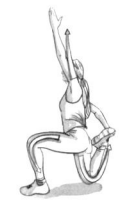

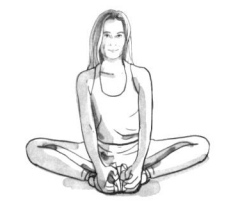

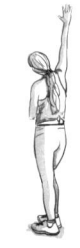

Done!

Note: we created a video timer specifically to guide you through your 4-3-2-1 workouts (especially when beginning) to help you get the hang of it. You can view these on the top left of each workout.

Each workout follows a 4-3-2-1 pattern; the specific exercises for each are described in detail in the workout index in the back of the book or via the Exercise Video Guide links listed on each workout page.

The four circuits in the actual workout will take you about 25 minutes to complete, including the warmup, cool-down, and **30-second break after each circuit**.

One day per week, the entire 4-3-2-1 workout will be dedicated to sculpting your butt and legs.

A second day of it will primarily aim to trim your waistline, develop your core, and strengthen your abdominal muscles.

A third day of it will have an ideal mix of lower body and upper body exercises for well-rounded muscle development and toning.

Why Use The '4-3-2-1' Method?

The 4-3-2-1 method is fundamentally rooted in *High Intensity Interval Training (HIIT)* which has been proven to torch the most fat as efficiently as possible.

Getting stronger and fitter is really a two-step process:

1. You need to do the strength training to build lean muscle mass, and
2. You need to do the right forms of cardiovascular exercise to burn body fat.

This dynamic duo will deliver the strong, badass body you want faster than any other approach (assuming you also stick with a healthy, protein-rich eating plan).

The good news is that the cardio part of the equation doesn't have to take over your life.

A 25 minute calorie-torching HIIT routine is the equivalent of 75 minutes of steady-paced cardio.

Who wouldn't want to save time and crush their fitness goals all at once?

The HIIT cardio approach embedded in the 4-3-2-1 method carries a whole bunch of specific health benefits like:

- It's the easiest way to lose belly fat while maintaining muscle mass
- Burn 3 times more calories than traditional cardiovascular workouts

- The 'After-Burn' effect causes your body to burn more calories for hours after your workout
- Chisels out your waist line
- Lowers fasting insulin and increases insulin sensitivity
- Boosts metabolism
- Improves HDL (the 'good' cholesterol)
- Reduces blood pressure
- Improves blood levels of health-protecting antioxidants

By alternating short bouts of high-intensity exercise with recovery intervals, HIIT gives you a huge bang for your buck, and it can be a fun change of pace from what you're currently accustomed to.

The main benefit of HIIT cardio over traditional cardio routines is '*the after-burn effect*' (Excess Post-Exercise Oxygen Consumption):

After any ordinary, steady-state cardio routine, your body takes about two hours to restore itself to pre-exercise levels, thus using more energy and burning excess calories for a few hours after your workout.

Because of the rigorous nature of HIIT workouts, the post-workout recovery demand on your body is greater and lasts longer. So, you naturally burn 15% more calories AFTER your workout than you would with an ordinary cardio routine.

In this way, we'll speed up the chiseling of your waist line by more quickly getting rid of the layer of fat around your belly.

Also, because of the nature of High Intensity Interval Training, you're targeting FAT loss rather than just losing calories.

Even more importantly, we'll be working towards building lean muscle mass *while* torching fat.

Resistance Training

The two remaining workouts in the week will consist of a variety of resistance training exercises to ensure that you're achieving the right muscle development to look as strong, fit, and sexy as possible!

We'll provide the exact exercises you should complete, the number of sets to do, and the number of reps to aim for.

Your job is to fill in the amount of weight you use (if you performed the workouts in a gym using weights, which is optional) and number of reps you actually completed in the designated tracking lines.

Why Resistance Training is Important

1. *It is the most effective way to build lean muscle*

For your tushy to transform into your optimal shape, you have to develop your glute muscles from all angles.

Simply put, resistance training causes the muscles to grow more quickly than other types of exercise because of the added resistance.

2. *The more lean muscle mass you have, the more calories you burn naturally throughout the day, leading to faster, better results.*

Your 'Basal Metabolic Rate' (**BMR**) is the number of calories you burn naturally throughout the day without exercise. This number is subject to fluctuation depending on a variety of factors. One of the big determining factors of your BMR is the amount of lean muscle mass you have. The more lean muscle mass in your body, the higher the rate at which it burns calories naturally!

3. *A big component of looking 'fit' is having the right proportion and symmetry of the upper half of your body in relation to the lower half of your body.*

When your upper back and shoulders are strong and toned, your waist automatically looks smaller, giving you what fitness enthusiasts call the 'V' shape—otherwise known as *The V-Line Taper*.

Each exercise in this program was deliberately chosen to give you this exact look.

NOTE: *For the two rest days during the week, feel free to choose how to use them! You can take the whole weekend off or just take breaks throughout the week as needed.*

The Pyramid Set Structure for Resistance Training

On resistance training days, we'll be using a 'Pyramid Set' structure. That means means we'll progressively be *increasing the weight* while *lowering the number of reps* as we move from set to set. Here's how it works:

On the first set of the exercise, you'll complete 10-15 repetitions. You should choose the amount of weight accordingly so that you can complete about 10-15 repetitions while still struggling at the end of the set.

On the second set of the same exercise, you'll increase the amount of weight you use, but only complete 8-10 reps of that exercise.

The same idea applies to the third and fourth sets for each exercise.

If you're doing the resistance training workouts at home without weights, then you should do the exercise to failure - as many repetitions as possible!

There are many benefits to pyramid sets. Possibly the biggest benefit is that there is essentially a built-in warm up on the first set that allows the muscle to prepare for heavier lifting. The lower rep range sets also give you a taste of what you're capable of. The amount of discomfort you face in your last few sets shows you how far you've come along.

When you can complete your last few sets with relative comfort and ease, you know it's time to move up in weight with all four sets! Pyramid sets force you to really test the limits of the muscle being worked. This leads to a greater understanding of your progress.

Resting Periods Between Sets

It is important to pay attention to how much rest you take in between sets. You need to give your muscles enough time to be ready for the next set while making sure you're not wasting time and are working with *maximum intensity*.

You'll need to find the proper balance for yourself. Your resting periods will decrease the more experienced you become.

In general, 30 seconds - 90 seconds in between sets is a good bench mark. Anything under may be too short, and anything over is probably too long. What's important is that you learn to recognize when you're wasting time out of laziness and to limit that as much as possible!

At Home Workouts: Alternative Exercises for Resistance Training Days

Almost every workout in this journal can be done at home, but as explained above, there are two resistance training days a week.

On these days, having access to a gym can be helpful, but it's definitely not required.

One option is buying just a couple of dumbbells and an elastic band with handles on it - that's basically all the equipment you need.

Whether or not you use this journal, dumbbells and an elastic resistance band are great to have around the house in case you ever want to exercise a little bit.

A second option if you don't want to spend extra money is to get creative with using at-home items to assist your workout and provide resistance for yourself.

- So many items around the house can be used as weights, such as water bottles.

- Stools, chairs, and couches can be used as platforms to step on.

- Towels and t-shirts can be used for resistance when being pulled between the hands.

- Lastly, you could simply flex your muscles tightly as you perform a movement to provide built-in resistance.

If you type into Google the name of a resistance training exercise that's in the journal and type 'at home version' at the end of it, you will get a bunch of alternative exercises to do.

Alternatively, if you encounter an exercise you aren't able to find proper alternatives for, you can email us directly at support@habitnest.com and ask for help, we'll do our best to give you suggestions for it.

The Two Primary Factors That Determine Your Progress

The truth of the matter is that trimming your waist, shaping your butt, and burning the necessary fat for your body to look great boils down to *two factors:*

1. Your diet
2. Doing the right type of exercise

We have you 100% covered when it comes to the proper exercise routine.

However, the effort and attention you give your diet needs to be your primary focus if you want to see the best results as quickly as possible.

Your diet provides the foundation for almost everything your body does, and it's central to any healthy fitness program.

Plus, what you eat provides the fuel for your workouts and the soothing salve for your body's post-exercise recovery. Using nutritious foods as sources of fuel, energy, and vitality will help you build lean, sculpted muscle, a healthy, resilient physique, and an overall badass body.

Optimizing Every Aspect of Your Nutrition

Some Basic Fat Loss Science

Note: Before following any nutrition advice in this journal, we recommend reaching out to your doctor and/or nutritionist to get their thoughts. Different people have different needs and it's always a good idea to check with a qualified professional about yours.

Achieving a Caloric Deficit

It's simple.

Your body needs a certain amount of energy to function.

A *calorie* is a unit of energy – it is the energy value of food.

When your body uses more calories than you're eating, it is forced to turn to other places to supply and fulfill the energy requirements it isn't getting from the food you're eating.

But the body has a few options for where it can go to take the energy that it needs. It can either go to fat stores, muscle protein, or a combination of both.

Our goal is to cause the body to use fat as its primary energy source.

When there is a caloric deficit and the body is forced to turn to alternate sources of energy, it is imperative to ensure that muscle catabolism doesn't occur.

Muscle catabolism is where your body uses muscle tissue for energy that it's not getting from the food you're eating.

To put everything into perspective, the moment you have a caloric surplus (you eat more calories than you burn), extra calories are stored as fat for future energy in the event that the body needs the energy later on.

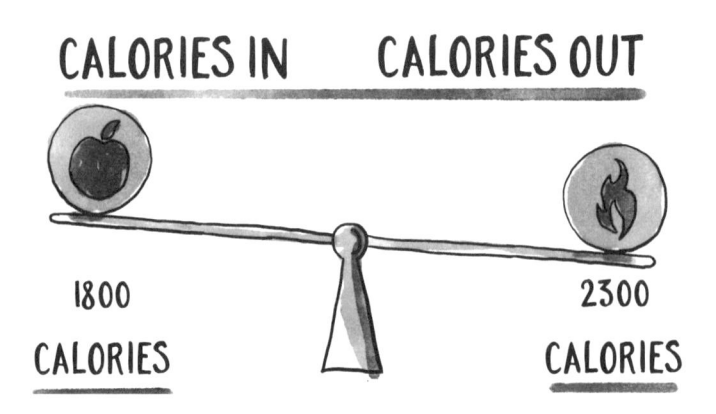

CALORIES IN — 1800 CALORIES

CALORIES OUT — 2300 CALORIES

Macronutrient Ratios

To lose weight, you need to eat less calories than you burn.[1] But to cause the body to specifically burn fat, you need to **understand how the macronutrients you eat affect your body**.

The term **macronutrient** refers to the main types of food – carbohydrates, lipids (fats), and proteins.

The macronutrient ratio refers to the percentage of your caloric intake of each of these three types of foods (how much you're eating from the different food groups).

To attain the right balance that will force your body to use fat for energy while retaining muscle, your macronutrient intake has to be carefully plotted and it must be tailored to your specific body type, the speed of your metabolism, and your ordinary activity levels.

In Summary:

1. Your body needs energy to function, and is in a constant state of energy expenditure.
2. A calorie is a unit of stored energy; a measure of the value of food.
3. You can force your body to burn fat by achieving a caloric deficit.
4. A caloric deficit results where you burn more calories than you consume.
5. A caloric deficit may result in your body using muscle tissue for energy, which we can prevent with a proper balance of macronutrients.

Carbohydrates
A Double-Edged Sword

We need energy to live. We need energy to breathe, to digest, to circulate blood flow, to move our limbs, to think, etc. From the moment we're born until the moment we leave this beautiful world, we are using energy to facilitate our every physical movement, thought, emotion and instinctive process.

Fat loss is really about re-directing the source of that energy by manipulating the body through the foods we eat.

---

[1] https://sciencebasedmedicine.org/calories-in-calories-out/

The body is extremely efficient. We have a very specific process for the way we create energy based on the food we eat. When there's an excess of what is needed, the body stores it to be used in a later day.

By the same token, when there's not enough energy supply, the body adapts and finds other sources.

Carbohydrates are the body's preferred source of energy.

Carbohydrates are vital to the functioning of our bodily systems. Carbs are broken down into glucose in the body. *Glucose* is the primary molecule that serves as energy for animals like us.

The main objective in achieving fat loss is forcing your body to react to circumstances you create by *using fat for energy rather than carbohydrates or muscle* tissue. We want our bodies to metabolize the fat that has been stored.[2]

That happens when you don't have enough carbohydrates in your system to supply all of your energy needs, so your body releases a hormone called **glucagon**, whose job is to convert existing fat that has been stored in the body into energy the body can use.

Glycogen refers to carbs that have been stored in the body. If you're continually eating carbs, which is the favored energy source, your body has absolutely no reason to metabolize fat for energy!

What's more is that when you eat more carbs than your body needs, the excess carbohydrates that can't currently be used as energy **are stored as fat**[3] so that they can potentially be used down the line if it becomes necessary.

A big part of fat loss is about regulating your carbohydrate intake to cause this bodily reaction of using fat as a source of energy.

But eliminating carbs completely is the wrong way to approach the task. Although it will help you achieve weight loss, you need to make sure your body isn't forced to reach for muscle tissue as the alternate supply of energy.

Carbohydrates are truly a double-edged sword.

---

[2] https://www.webmd.com/diabetes/type-1-diabetes-guide/what-is-ketosis#1

[3] https://www.ncsf.org/enew/articles/articles-convertingcarbs.aspx

Although eliminating carbs does lead to the using of fat and muscle as alternate energy supplies, eating carbs **protects muscle tissue**, thereby forcing the burning of fat rather than muscle.[4]

*The balance is a **real** struggle*:

Too many carbs and your body won't burn fat. Too little carbs, and your body burns through your muscle tissue. But, don't worry. Soon you'll have everything you need to find the right balance for your body.

Quality of Carbs

There are two main types of carbohydrates, commonly referred to as '**simple carbs**' and '**complex carbs**.' What defines the quality of a carbohydrate is the speed at which it is absorbed – the rate at which your body breaks them down for use as energy.

Simple Carbohydrates

When carbohydrates are absorbed quickly (when simple carbohydrates are consumed), there is a quick bodily reaction of elevated blood sugar, which causes the brain to release the hormone **insulin** to get the body's blood sugar levels back under control.

The resulting danger is that when insulin is set in motion to regulate blood sugar, the hormone glucagon (the hormone that asks the body to use fat as an energy supply) is halted until the insulin has finished its work. Your body regulates the blood sugar while fat burning is suppressed.

Another common negative attribute of 'simple' or *fast-absorbing carbohydrates* is that giving your body that high elevation in blood sugar results in an equally low swing in the opposite direction. Basically, after insulin kicks in and lowers your blood sugar, then your body craves food to push it back up.

You feel hungry quickly.
The long-term result is a complete loss of control in the way we handle our food. We over-eat, and we crave the same unhealthy carbohydrates that gave us the rush in the first place.

Regulating your carbohydrate intake is largely about regulating blood sugar levels to keep them at a balanced level.

---

[4] https://www.ncbi.nlm.nih.gov/pmc/articles/PMC1373635/

Some examples of simple carbohydrates are: Baked goods, cookies, sugar, cereal, corn syrup, fruit juice concentrate, and dairy products.

Complex Carbohydrates

Complex carbohydrates are those that cause smaller increases in blood sugar because they take more time for the body to break down and use (they have longer chains of sugar molecules). They allow glucose to release into the blood stream slowly and consistently.

You want to fill as much of your carbohydrate intake with complex carbohydrates as possible.

Some great complex carbs are brown rice, whole wheat bread, yams, broccoli, carrots, pasta, quinoa, grains, beans, and fiber-rich fruits.

Fiber is an interesting complex carbohydrate worth noting because it slows down the rate at which your body absorbs other types of carbohydrates. Fiber is also indigestible, meaning that your body completely gets rid of it after its been made proper use of.

The Glycemic Index

The glycemic index is a scale that rates foods that can be categorized as carbohydrates based on the effect in the rise of blood sugar that the food has. Generally speaking, the higher the glycemic index rating (which is anywhere from 1 – 100), the more 'simple' the carbohydrate is.

To get the most out of the carbohydrates you consume, try checking where the carbs you eat fall on this scale. The goal is to eat foods that fall ideally from 1-40 on the scale the majority of the time, and 40-75 sparingly.

GLYCEMIC INDEX CHART
LOW GLYCEMIC (55 OR BELOW)   HIGH GLYCEMIC (70 OR HIGHER)

SNACKS	G.I.	STARCH	G.I.	VEGETABLES	G.I.	FRUITS	G.I.	DAIRY	G.I.
PIZZA	33	BAGEL, PLAIN	33	BROCCOLI	10	CHERRIES	22	YOGURT, PLAIN	14
CHOCOLATE BAR	49	WHITE RICE	38	PEPPER	10	APPLE	38	YOGURT, LOW FAT	14
POUND CAKE	54	WHITE SPAGHETTI	38	LETTUCE	10	ORANGE	43	WHOLE MILK	30
POPCORN	55	SWEET POTATO	44	MUSHROOMS	10	GRAPES	46	SOY MILK	31
ENERGY BAR	58	WHITE BREAD	49	ONIONS	10	KIWI	52	SKIM MILK	32
SODA	72	BROWN RICE	55	GREEN PEAS	48	BANANA	56	CHOCOLATE MILK	35
DOUGHNUT	76	PANCAKES	67	CARROTS	49	PINEAPPLE	66	YOGURT, FRUIT	36
JELLY BEANS	80	WHEAT BREAD	80	BEETS	64	WATERMELON	72	CUSTARD	43
PRETZELS	83	BAKED POTATO	85			DATES	103	ICE CREAM	60

In Summary:

1. Eliminating carbs is not the answer to a great body, although it can help you achieve rapid weight loss.

2. The body prefers carbohydrates as its main source of energy. Carbohydrates are converted into glucose and used as energy for bodily functions and processes.

3. You can cause your body to use fat and protein as a source of energy by regulating your carbohydrate intake.

4. Carbohydrates protect your muscle tissue from being used as energy, so it is important to find the right portion of carbohydrates to eat.

5. Simple carbohydrates cause rapid increases in blood sugar, which stops your body from burning fat and leaves you feeling hungry.

6. Fill your carbohydrate intake with complex carbohydrates like yams, brown rice, whole wheat bread, grains, vegetables, quinoa, fiber-rich fruits, and beans.

7. The glycemic index rates the complexity of carbohydrates based on the way they affect blood sugar levels after consumption.

8. The lower on the glycemic index scale a carbohydrate falls, the better it is for fat loss.

Proteins

You have over 10,000 different proteins in your body. Protein is absolutely essential to every cell in the body. It is made up of amino acids, which, in relation to weight loss, are important in that they **grow and repair our muscle tissue**.

It is essential to consume enough protein because it helps keep you full, stimulates muscle growth, facilitates muscle retention, and it has a significant affect on our basal metabolic rate – the automatic functioning of our metabolism.[5]

The more protein you eat, the faster your metabolism works. The faster your metabolism works, the more calories you naturally burn.

The mechanics of the way protein affects the metabolism are relatively simple.

If paired with exercise, protein enlarges muscles by adding additional proteins to muscle fibers. That process requires amino acids. When you eat more amino acids, which are what protein is made up of, it has a direct affect on muscle mass.

Increasing your muscle mass has an affect on the amount of calories you naturally burn because muscle tissue requires more energy than fat.

The more muscle you have and the less fat present in your body, the faster your metabolism operates.[6]

It's been said a few times already that fat loss is achieved by forcing the body to burn fat as a result of a caloric deficit. We've also said that the body turns not only to fat, but to muscle when it has energy requirements it needs to fulfill.

Although eating a certain amount of carbohydrates can curb the use of muscle tissue as an energy source, it is really important to continue to fill the body with protein to maintain the muscle in your body. Eating protein ensures that you continue to burn fat while keeping your muscle.

Another benefit of heavier protein consumption is that your body takes longer to digest, which requires the use of more energy in the process, and protein keeps you full for long periods of time.

Some great sources of protein include cottage cheese, eggs, steak, lean chicken, turkey, fish, beans, lentils, quinoa, protein and nuts.

---

[5] https://www.ncbi.nlm.nih.gov/pubmed/18448177; https://www.ncbi.nlm.nih.gov/pubmed/19640952

[6] https://www.ncbi.nlm.nih.gov/pmc/articles/PMC4258944/

Fats

Your body requires you to eat fat in order to burn fat. It is indispensable to eat some forms of healthy fats. **Essential fats** keep your skin and hair healthy, and are integral to hormone production.

'Good fats' are titled 'essential' because the body can't produce them on its own, or work properly without them. They're also important for brain development, and controlling inflammation in the body.

'Bad fats' or 'saturated/trans fats' have no true nutritional value and in fact harm the basic processes they're meant to help facilitate.

When you eat a lot of fat with (very) few carbohydrates, the metabolism changes and is placed into a state of **Ketosis**, which is another word to describe the process of burning fat rather than carbohydrates as an energy source.

Healthy fat consumption can come from vegetable oils, all sorts of nuts, avocados, eggs, chia seeds, fatty fish, coconuts (in addition to coconut oil), peanut butter, seeds, greek yogurt, and even dark chocolate.

In Summary:

1. The more protein you consume and fill your muscles with, the faster your metabolism works.
2. Protein helps to ensure that you will burn fat while retaining muscle.
3. Protein keeps you full for longer periods of time and keeps the digestive process active.
4. You need to eat fat to burn fat, but it's important to refrain from eating saturated fat or trans-fat.
5. Nuts are the easiest and best way to consume the fat you need in your diet.

Taking Action on Your Nutrition Goals

At this point, most people will take a mental note on these dietary / food points to apply going forward. But in order to **guarantee our results,** we must **guarantee we'll take action on this every day.**

As powerful as mindsets are, they are also very malleable and easily influenced by outside stimuli (like having a very common 'off day'). Meanwhile, systems (which provide accountability and tracking) are black and white - yes or no - 1 or 0.

We highly recommend putting together a structure you think can work in helping you stay consistent with your eating goals. Nothing is more demoralizing than aiming to feel better about yourself, working out hard for it, and seeing poor results (that you later justify).

After getting some clarity on which eating plan you want to follow (e.g. counting calories/macros or choosing a specific diet), there are a few ways to put it into effect.

As a free option

You can use a dietary tracking app, google sheet, or notepad to track calories/macros/meals. Alternatively you can use an extra whiteboard or calendar to track whether you hit your goals or not every day. If you think you can genuinely stay consistent with this for months / the long term, this is a great option.

As a paid option

Co-authors of this journal, Habit Nest, wrote the *The Nutrition Sidekick Journal* to help you nail down your diet - by providing a clear, unbreakable system to track your results and help you learn how to improve (without judgement!) at the same time.

If a pure tracking sheet is a bit too dull, redundant, and isn't stimulating enough for you, this may be the right choice.

Some things covered inside:

1. How to manipulate your body to burn fat while maintaining muscle
2. Tracking for your calories, water intake, and planned meals vs. actual eaten meals
3. New golden nuggets of information, pro-tips, daily challenges, and more each day

You can check it out at **SidekickJournal.com/Nutrition** and use discount code **BadassBooty15** for 15% off if you decide to order one.

Effectively Tracking Your Progress

Tracking your progress is extremely important. That being said, the accuracy of your tracking is **even more important**. With flawed data that isn't actionable, your tracking is just an arbitrary, confusing, and often misleading number.

This section assumes you have two body-composition goals, which tend to be the most popular amongst people (and can be the healthiest):

1. You want to increase your muscle mass
2. You want to reach & maintain your body fat percentage at 5-15% (males) or 10-20% (females)

If the above is true, as a general guideline your goal should first be to get as lean as you'd like, then switch to a *very slight* caloric surplus to build muscle in the long-term.

The problem with the scale

With resistance training and fat loss, the scale's results (without deeper insight on it) can be your biggest enemy. This is because our shifts in bodyweight are affected by SO many factors, it's impossible to identify what has changed week by week with only a weight amount.

This is where **body fat tracking** comes in, right alongside **body weight tracking**. By combining the tracking of BOTH your body fat AND the scale, you're able to see exactly HOW your weight changed from week to week - whether you gained muscle, gained body fat, lost muscle, or lost body fat.

Measuring your body fat percentage accurately

There are many ways to do this, but the most cost-effective and practical way is to use a self-testing skinfold caliper. The one we recommend is the Accu-Measure as it costs roughly $10 on Amazon and has an existing scientific study backing up its effectiveness (it's within 1.1% accuracy of using an underwater body fat measurement, which is one of the highest levels of accuracy we have for measuring body fat).

Disclaimer: We have no affiliation with the Accu-Measure and aren't getting paid in any way for this recommendation. It's simply a great tool.

With the upsides being ease of use and cost, the biggest downsides of this method are the **potential inaccuracy** if you don't know how to measure yourself properly each week. Although it's **very possible to be incredibly accurate** with this method… it takes a good deal of practice. Thankfully, the product comes with step-by-step guide that lays out how to use it as accurately as possible.

Even if your placement isn't perfect, as long as you are measuring yourself in the same location every week, you'll be able to have comparable results you trust week after week. Make your main goal in measuring be *consistency in measuring*.

How do I get the right data?

We recommend measuring yourself weekly for both body weight (with a scale) and body fat (with the Accu-Measure).

We want to eliminate as many factors that can cause data inconsistencies as possible. When taking your measurements, do it:

- At the same time of day (ideally mornings)
- With the same food/water intake that day (ideally none, do it right as you wake up)
- With the same amount of clothes on, and
- Without holding any objects that could throw your readings off (e.g. your phone)

You can write this data down as you progress through the journal (turn the page!) or record it on a note on your phone. If you choose the latter, make sure you don't hold your phone as you're measuring yourself.

Common misunderstandings with the Accu-Measure

After using the Accu-Measure ourselves, a few things were a bit unclear from the instruction sheet they provided. We spoke with a rep on the phone who helped clarify these points for us:

1. Where is the iliac crest?
To find your iliac crest, it should be near your waist line (like where you wear a belt) and you feel a big bone protruding out, towards the side of your body.

2. How can you measure consistently and accurately?
If you place the caliper directly on your skin, the ends will measure 2.5 inches exactly. You can use this to consistently grab the same distance each measurement.

Once you have grabbed your skin fold with your thumb and index finger, position the caliper halfway between the back of your skinfold (point closest to your body) and the front of the skinfold (point furthest from your body), 1cm away from your fingers.

Getting even more clarity, reducing measuring inaccuracy

The most important thing with using the Accu-Measure is **measuring yourself the same way week-to-week**. Even if you're measuring yourself improperly, or the Accu-Measure is inaccurate itself, your **week-to-week changes should remain consistent** as the method of measuring is consistent.

If you want to take this to the next level (or see how close to accurate your Accu-Measure is), you can get a detailed body scan (e.g. a $45 DEXA scan or water displacement scan) and see how it compares to the Accu-Measure. If a discrepancy exists, you'll at least know by how much and be able to mentally keep that in mind.

Write down the following each week

1. Measure your **total body weight** using a scale

2. Measure your **body fat %** using an Accu-Measure

3. Take your total body weight (#1) in pounds and multiply it by your body fat % (#2). This will give you your **body fat weight**.

4. Take your **total body weight** (#1) and subtract your **body fat weight** (#3) to get your **lean body mass**.

Your lean body mass consists of every part of your body that's not considered fat (muscles, tissues, bones, organs, water weight, etc.) Since a significant changing factor in weight of your lean body mass is your muscle mass, we can use lean body mass as a near-accurate measure of fluctuations in muscle gain / loss.

The biggest inconsistency with your lean body mass will be the fluctuations in your water weight. Be mindful of this and how certain factors (e.g. being dehydrated, drinking lots of water, intaking too much sodium the day before) can affect this. If something seems wrong, give it at least 2 weeks before jumping to conclusions of whether your plan is or is not working.

What should I do with this measurement data?

The next two pages provide a space to record this data weekly over a 12-week period, followed by actions steps for how to adjust weekly for each scenario.

Having this data recorded next to each other will allow you to spot trends in your weekly fluctuations and make the correct adjustments of action steps based on this.

Adjusting Based on Your Progress

As recommended in Tom Venuto's *Burn The Fat, Feed The Muscle*, you should make the following tweaks based on your weekly fluctuations of **body fat weight (B.F. Weight)** and **lean body mass (L.B.M.)**[7] to achieve body fat loss & muscle gain:

1. *If:* [B.F. Weight ↑]   [L.B.M. ↑]

Then: Decrease your caloric intake (recommended: 100-200) and increase your cardio.

2. *If:* [B.F. Weight ↓]   [L.B.M. ↑]

Then: This is the holy grail and we are all jealous of you. Keep doing what you're doing. This is decently rare to occur, so treat it as a huge gift if you're lucky to experiencing it!

3. *If:* [B.F. Weight ↑]   [L.B.M. ↓]

Then: This is unlikely and usually due to a measurement inaccuracy. Alternatively, this may be due to factors outside of your training and nutrition, such as being under a lot of stress and not getting adequate rest. Recheck your results, and if they're accurate, take care of yourself and see if you notice a significant difference the following week.

4. *If:* [B.F. Weight ↓]   [L.B.M. ↓]

Then: Eat more calories (recommended: 100-200) and increase protein intake if you're under 1g * your total body weight.
Increasing your resistance training intensity will help as well here.

5. *If:* [B.F. Weight ↑]   [L.B.M. —]   (This icon means "stayed the same.")

Then: Eat less calories (recommended: 100-200) and slightly increase your cardio.
Note: This action step also applies if both your L.B.M. and your body fat weight stay the same (no change as the week before).

6. *If:* [B.F. Weight ↓]   [L.B.M. —]

Then: This is fantastic! You're right on track, keep doing what you're doing.

---

[7] https://en.wikipedia.org/wiki/Lean_body_mass

Weekly Progress Tracker

WEEK 1

DATE: _____

WEIGHT: _____   BODY FAT %: _____

FAT WEIGHT: _____   LEAN BODY MASS: _____

ADJUSTMENTS TO MAKE
(CIRCLE)   (FILL IN AMOUNT)

CALORIES   ↑   ↓   —   _____

CARDIO   ↑   ↓   —   _____

TRAINING INTENSITY   ↑   ↓   —

WEEK 2

DATE: _____

WEIGHT: _____   BODY FAT %: _____

FAT WEIGHT: _____   LEAN BODY MASS: _____

ADJUSTMENTS TO MAKE
(CIRCLE)   (FILL IN AMOUNT)

CALORIES   ↑   ↓   —   _____

CARDIO   ↑   ↓   —   _____

TRAINING INTENSITY   ↑   ↓   —

WEEK 3

DATE: _____

WEIGHT: _____   BODY FAT %: _____

FAT WEIGHT: _____   LEAN BODY MASS: _____

ADJUSTMENTS TO MAKE
(CIRCLE)   (FILL IN AMOUNT)

CALORIES   ↑   ↓   —   _____

CARDIO   ↑   ↓   —   _____

TRAINING INTENSITY   ↑   ↓   —

WEEK 4

DATE: _____

WEIGHT: _____   BODY FAT %: _____

FAT WEIGHT: _____   LEAN BODY MASS: _____

ADJUSTMENTS TO MAKE
(CIRCLE)   (FILL IN AMOUNT)

CALORIES   ↑   ↓   —   _____

CARDIO   ↑   ↓   —   _____

TRAINING INTENSITY   ↑   ↓   —

WEEK 5

DATE: _____

WEIGHT: _____   BODY FAT %: _____

FAT WEIGHT: _____   LEAN BODY MASS: _____

ADJUSTMENTS TO MAKE
(CIRCLE)   (FILL IN AMOUNT)

CALORIES   ↑   ↓   —   _____

CARDIO   ↑   ↓   —   _____

TRAINING INTENSITY   ↑   ↓   —

WEEK 6

DATE: _____

WEIGHT: _____   BODY FAT %: _____

FAT WEIGHT: _____   LEAN BODY MASS: _____

ADJUSTMENTS TO MAKE
(CIRCLE)   (FILL IN AMOUNT)

CALORIES   ↑   ↓   —   _____

CARDIO   ↑   ↓   —   _____

TRAINING INTENSITY   ↑   ↓   —

WEEK 7

DATE: _____

WEIGHT: _____   BODY FAT %: _____

FAT WEIGHT: _____   LEAN BODY MASS: _____

ADJUSTMENTS TO MAKE
(CIRCLE)   (FILL IN AMOUNT)

CALORIES   ↑   ↓   —   _____

CARDIO   ↑   ↓   —   _____

TRAINING INTENSITY ↑   ↓   —

WEEK 8

DATE: _____

WEIGHT: _____   BODY FAT %: _____

FAT WEIGHT: _____   LEAN BODY MASS: _____

ADJUSTMENTS TO MAKE
(CIRCLE)   (FILL IN AMOUNT)

CALORIES   ↑   ↓   —   _____

CARDIO   ↑   ↓   —   _____

TRAINING INTENSITY ↑   ↓   —

WEEK 9

DATE: _____

WEIGHT: _____   BODY FAT %: _____

FAT WEIGHT: _____   LEAN BODY MASS: _____

ADJUSTMENTS TO MAKE
(CIRCLE)   (FILL IN AMOUNT)

CALORIES   ↑   ↓   —   _____

CARDIO   ↑   ↓   —   _____

TRAINING INTENSITY ↑   ↓   —

WEEK 10

DATE: _____

WEIGHT: _____   BODY FAT %: _____

FAT WEIGHT: _____   LEAN BODY MASS: _____

ADJUSTMENTS TO MAKE
(CIRCLE)   (FILL IN AMOUNT)

CALORIES   ↑   ↓   —   _____

CARDIO   ↑   ↓   —   _____

TRAINING INTENSITY ↑   ↓   —

Getting Started

Goal-Setting Principles

Whether you're working towards fitness goals or other personal goals to improve the quality of your life, the process of creating a lasting change is multi-faceted.

It boils down to:

1. Having a concrete goal you want to reach,
2. Creating a realistic action plan that'll take you towards your goal,
3. Preparing mentally and emotionally for obstacles that will undoubtedly arise,
4. Utilizing a proper system of accountability,
5. Tracking your progress so you see the results and benefits you're gaining, and
6. Taking action daily.

In terms of creating the action plan, using a system of accountability, tracking your progress, and discussing many of the obstacles that will arise, we have you covered from A-Z.

But, even though the entire blueprint is laid out, nothing changes without your daily action and commitment to your goal!

Your brain has to change before your body can.

Why We Know This Program Works

Fitness and performance expert Jennifer Cohen, co-author of this book and bestselling author of *Strong Is The New Skinny* and *No Gym Required* has trained hundreds of clients using the training method you're given here.

Even more importantly, she is an entrepreneur involved in several businesses and a mother of two.

Jen continues to find the time every day to implement this routine to keep herself in great shape.

The program has been intricately designed to combat the results of our bodies storing fat in our stomachs, hips, thighs, and butts, and re-shaping these problem areas to achieve a toned, fit look.

Perfectionists, Tread Lightly.

In a perfect (and very imaginary) world, we all want to work out consistently and see the results as soon as we begin a new exercise regimen.

But sometimes there's a problem with shooting for perfection from the very start.

So often you see people getting caught up in finding "the best workout routine," or "the best diet for weight loss" that they never end up acting on their goal.

But we're going to let you in on a little secret.

There's one simple concept that shatters all the best research, tips and strategies you can look for (that you'll be getting here anyways).

The best way to shape your booty and trim your waist to get those amazing results is…. to start and do something.

You start taking SOME action towards your goal on a daily basis.

Don't let the desire to reach perfection - your goal body - stop you from making sure you have a great workout TODAY.

The best way to get the body you want is by trying one method for achieving it; following one specific strategy that has been laid out and doing it consistently for a period of time.

Nobody else can do your workouts for you. All they can do is give you information.

It's up to YOU to try the program, learn what you can, see how effective it is, and only then make an educated choice about how to move forward.

You'll be getting all the information and motivation you need from us on a daily basis in the workouts you're getting.

If you make use of every workout to just take a small step towards your goal, you WILL see the results you're after. Pinky promise.

Because every little action you take in the direction of your goals propels a snowball effect that greatly impacts other areas of your life.

If you push yourself to do this program for even 1 week, you're gifting yourself a positive chain of effects that will improve your daily energy, mental clarity, and increase your self-confidence.

In turn, if you don't prioritize your workouts, each of these benefits gets sacrificed.

Break through every obstacle you may face to absolutely get your workout done TODAY.

And then repeat.

Because success is all about taking small, consistent actions over time.

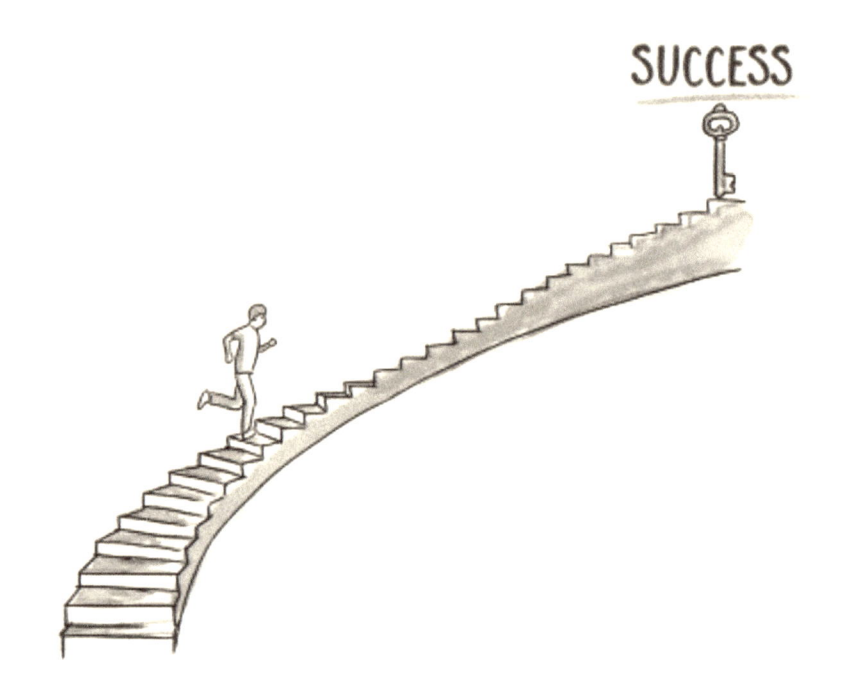

Holding Yourself Accountable
Staying Consistent

One of the best ways to continue doing this habit is to build it alongside a friend who is also passionate about becoming the best version of themself. Having someone to talk to and brainstorm about your specific pain points makes a huge difference. Their support (and sometimes competitive kick) can serve as a nice backup too.

Whether or not that person is also using this journal alongside you, you're still able to work together on establishing a consistent habit together.

If you're the type of person who benefits from a sense of community, we created a free Facebook group specifically designed to hold yourself accountable to using this journal, getting daily support, and for building habits in general.

There's daily activity on there and our team is extremely involved each day.

Join the Habit Nest accountability group here:
facebook.com/groups/habitnest

Developing Strength From the Inside Out

Your head can be your friend or foe when it comes to getting stronger, fitter, and sexier.

That's because your mind is your most powerful muscle, so you can either flex it to boost your motivation and perseverance (which is great) or clench it to resist your efforts (which is bad).

Our advice is to pick option number one.

Here is what you stand to gain: A stronger, more consistent sense of motivation, a can-do spirit, a clearer vision of your goals and the mental clarity and fortitude to reach them.

So ask yourself: is your mind your ally or enemy when it comes to getting fit?

When you think about your body - its state, its shape, and its capabilities - do your thoughts sound more like the captain of your own cheerleading squad or more like an abusive schoolyard bully?

If it's the latter, it's time to evict that critical, sadistic voice and replace it with a more positive one.

The key is to change the way you think and talk about your body; if you don't have anything nice to say, shut up already!

Seriously, it's time to reclaim your mind and put it to good use for your body's sake.

If you've already got an upbeat mind, you can kick up your mental strength and positivity a notch or two and take it to the next level.

The truth is that you can talk yourself into or out of anything, so why not steer yourself in a positive direction?

Cranking up the strength in your head while you're ramping up your physical strength will produce a win-win outcome:

The mental vigor you'll be developing will fuel your physical fitness and vice versa, creating an awesome mind-body synergy that will help you grow and thrive and become the best version of yourself yet.

When you condition your body to overcome hurdles or bounce back from setbacks, you will encourage your mind to do the same. It's a two-way street.

You Are Perfect as You Are

In going through this process, it's crucial to keep in mind that you are already perfect and that increasing your confidence and becoming a healthier you has nothing to do with your innate quality as a human being.

Looking or not looking a certain way does not make you inferior or superior to anyone else. Exercise and healthy eating are essential parts of living a well-rounded, healthy life.

They are objectively related to your health, well-being and weight loss.

Your end goal here isn't to be a certain weight or look a certain way, **it's to increase the quality of your emotional relationship with yourself**. You want to increase your energy levels, confidence, acceptance and ultimately love for yourself.

Never forget that changing your body through exercise and diet is simply a vehicle for that. If you can get there regardless of food, you've won the true battle.

What Are You Waiting For?

Everybody knows what their personal best is, and if you are not there or anywhere near it in terms of looking and feeling the way you want to, you have to ask yourself, "What am I waiting for?"

You (hopefully) just learned a lot about booty-building, torching fat through exercise and diet, and how we're going to help you attain your fitness goals.

But even though the blueprint for the plan is completely laid out and you have all the tools you need for hitting your goal, you have to remember that this whole process starts and ends **with you**.

Your job is to commit to the plan - mentally, physically, and emotionally until you realize that you can and will reach your goal with the right attitude.

With an attitude that is dead-set on reaching the goal you set out to accomplish, literally nothing can stop you.

The Three Factors of Behavior Change

James Clear, author of *Atomic Habits*, writes that there's essentially three parts to behavior change (we love your work, James!).

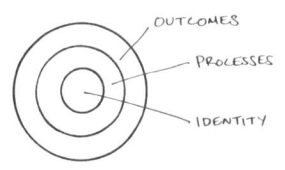

1. The Outcomes

The first is the outside layer, the outcomes. This is synonymous with your goals or where you want to get to, e.g. I want to achieve 15% body fat and have visible abs.

Outcomes are most useful at setting a larger, over-arching vision for where you want to go to. The downsides of over-focusing on your outcomes are relying on hitting your goals to bring you happiness instead of enjoying the process, and a lack of practicality for what to do day-to-day.

Your outcomes are likely to change over the course of your life to match your ever-evolving goals and needs.

2. The Processes

The second, middle layer, is about processes — this boils down to what system and action steps you put in place to make your outcomes come to be. These are things like I will work out 4 times a week, I will try to increase the reps and/or the speed of an exercise each time. Synonymous with strategies and tactics.

These can be very useful, especially when you find one that clicks, and you'll see a number for you to experiment with sprinkled throughout the journal.

These processes are likely to change over time as you test different ones out, see what works best for you, and switch things up when you get bored / desensitized to them.

3a. Your Identity

This one's the big kahuna. This is the inner-most layer, matching who your internal belief is of yourself as a person. The biggest mistake people make in enacting behavior change is placing way too large of a focus on the first two parts of this puzzle, while entirely forgetting about the third and the most impactful — how you view yourself.

By properly emphasizing WHO you want to grow into, you will maximize your self-respect, satisfaction, and ability to control your actions — more than any motivation or strategy can give you. Your identity is what you can always fall back to set your intuition, to guide you to what you should really be doing.

An example of setting your identity is:

"I'm someone who does what it take to get lean, fit, strong, and healthy. I do what's right, not what's easy, in working out and staying consistent with my nutrition and fitness goals."

> *After defining the identity you want to grow into for yourself, chances are this will **not change much**, but rather, only **strengthen over time** based on your actions.*

3b. Your Identity On Your Off-Days

As much as this plays a role in building towards your goals, it's equally as important in regards to times where you fall off the wagon.

Most people subconsciously forget about what their self-identity looks like when this happens, allowing a massive negative self-view to kick in.

This leads to a major emotional factor, *guilt*, to kick in, and as many studies have shown, **guilt is a willpower destroyer** (these are cited at the end of the book).

Instead, mindfully set your identity in these situations. We have two recommendations for this:

> Grow into the person who uses every opportunity of falling off-track to further strengthen your ability to *switch from your off-days back to being on-track.*

Chances are you won't have perfect consistency with your nutrition and fitness, every single day, for the rest of your life, right? Life is about knowing which habits to employ, at the right time, to help you get the most fulfillment out of life.

This involves testing different things and seeing how they serve your life's purpose. In order to really do this, you must master the ability to switch back and forth and how to quickly rebuild the momentum you had with your habits, without any guilt that you "lost your mojo."

Be the type of person who can forgive yourself for your mistakes, who will love yourself unconditionally and be a true best friend to yourself (because if you can't, who will?)

We know these are big emphases on emotional states that can come off "fluffy" but the truth is our fulfillment in life directly ties to our emotional states. Learning how to master them is the true feat of this journal, not just building up a specific habit.

Establishing Your Identity

Write your identity statement here.

What kind of person do you want to grow into through this process?

_____
_____
_____
_____

What kind of person do you want to be when you fall off the wagon of your habits? What do you want to remember about who you are and how you can repurpose these days to serve your life?

_____
_____
_____
_____

General Safety Tips

For All Days:
1. If you begin feeling any pain, do NOT continue with an exercise. Feel free to switch to any exercise that does not cause you pain.

2. You always want the muscle you're working on to take the load, not your back or other parts of the body - all it takes is ONE bad set, ONE bad rep to set you back weeks, or even months.

3. Don't extend to the absolute limit of your flexibility unless you're extremely comfortable with the exercise.

4. Be aware of your surroundings. Make sure there's nothing you could knock over or could injure you during your workouts, especially those with movement.

For Resistance Training Days:
1. Never invent new uses for a machine!

2. When picking up weights, use proper form. Bend with your knees and use leg strength to pick up the weight (as opposed to using your back or hips).

3. If you're unsure whether or not you can complete a rep without just dropping the weights, USE a ***spotter*** - someone to help you finish the movement if you get stuck.

4. Don't just drop weights, they fall hard and bounce around. You can hurt others or yourself when you drop the weights from your hands to the floor. Use a controlled movement to place weights on the ground or in their proper place.

5. Fingers and toes are weirdly susceptible to getting hurt when picking up or putting weights down - watch out for it. Our cofounder Ari once bruised his finger because he put the weight on the rack too quickly and the dumbbell went over the rack with his finger caught in between it and the rack.

6. If you've made the very normal mistake of using a weight that's too heavy for you and you realize you need help because you're in a situation in which you're not sure what to do - ASK for help from somebody nearby!!

7. Always be aware of your surroundings - make sure what you're doing doesn't jeopardize anybody else's safety.

8. If using at-home alternatives, always put safety first and consider how an object may fall out of place or put you in danger. We recommend only using stable, static objects that cannot slide, slip, or injure you in any way.

The Extreme Importance of Form

Before beginning any exercise, you have to be absolutely sure that you understand how to complete the exercise properly without getting injured.

We provide explanations of each exercise in the back of this journal, but if you're ever unclear, it only takes 30 seconds to look any exercise up online.

Our bodies are masters of compensation.

Where the body can 'cheat' by using more muscles than necessary to complete a movement, it will.

There must be a constant vigilance to retain proper form. And let's be very clear: Form is **vitally** important.

<u>Without proper form</u>:

1. There is always a *risk of injury.*
2. You're most likely *missing the target muscle* because you're *overcompensating with body parts that don't need to be used.*

There is never a good reason not to use proper form on any given exercise.

Commit.

No matter what happens tomorrow...

*whether I am exhausted
or have the **worst** day of my life...*

*...whether I win the lottery
or have the **best** day of my life...*

I <u>will</u> do my workout.

*My word is like **gold.***

*I will do whatever it takes
to make this happen.*

I will workout at least this many times this week (circle one):

1   2   3   4   5   6   7

_____   _____
Signature   Date

The Workouts

EXERCISE GUIDE
https://HabitNest.link/booty01

Workout 1: 4-3-2-1

GLUTE ACTIVATION WARMUP
30s EACH

a. Clam Opener

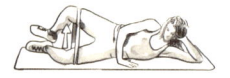

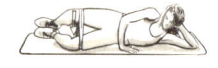

(30s Each Leg)

b. Glute Bridge w/ Band Flutter

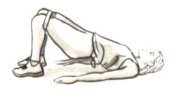

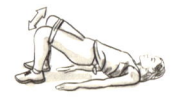

c. Fire Hydrant

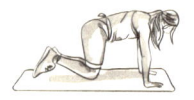

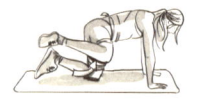

(30s Each Side)

d. Lateral Leg Raise

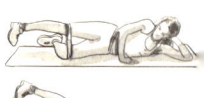

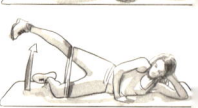

- 30s Each Leg (w/ Foot Flexed)
- 30s Each Leg (w/ Toes Pointing)

(Note: Refer to the Exercise Index the back of this book if you nee further clarification on how to perform any of these exercises

--- 30 SECOND BREAK ---

CIRCUIT 1
60s EACH

1a. Curtsy Lunge

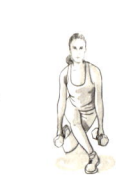

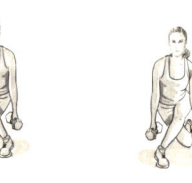

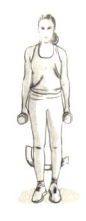

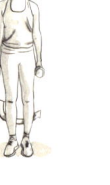

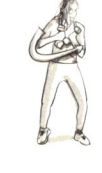

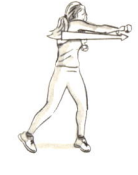

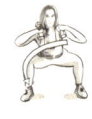

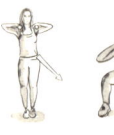

REPS: _____
(Left Leg)

→

1b. Curtsy Lunge

REPS: _____
(Right Leg)

→

1c. Boxing Jab

REPS: _____

→

1d. Side to Side Squat

REPS: _____

--- 30 SECOND BREAK ---

CIRCUIT 2
50s EACH

2a. 180° Jump Twist to Floor Tap

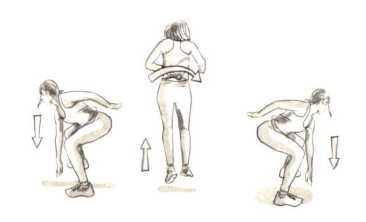

SET 1 REPS: _____
SET 2 REPS: _____

→

2b. Squat to Overhead Press

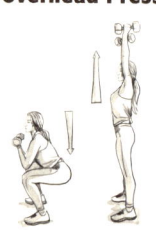

SET 1 REPS: _____
SET 2 REPS: _____

→

2c. Plie Jump Squat

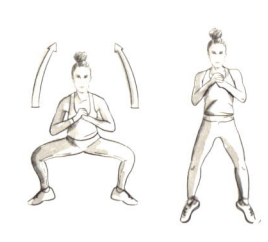

SET 1 REPS: _____
SET 2 REPS: _____

--- 30 SECOND BREAK ---

CIRCUIT 3
40s EACH

3a. Lateral Lunge to Reverse Lunge

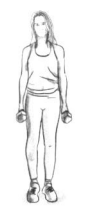

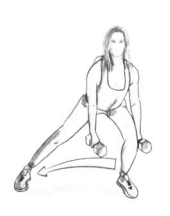

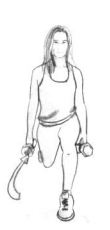

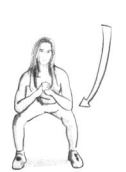

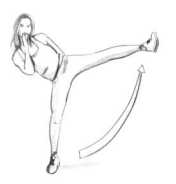

(Left Leg)   SET 1 REPS: _____   →
(Right Leg)   SET 2 REPS: _____   →
(Alternate Legs) SET 3 REPS: _____   →

3b. Roundhouse Kick to Squat

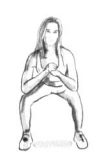

(Left Leg)   SET 1 REPS: _____
(Right Leg)   SET 2 REPS: _____
(Alternate Legs) SET 3 REPS: _____

--- 30 SECOND BREAK ---

4a. Leap Forward into Squat, Burpee, Shuffle Back

CIRCUIT 4
30s EACH

(Reminder: If you feel pain with any exercise, STOP! Do NOT push through. Try a different exercise instead.)

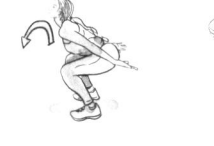

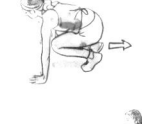

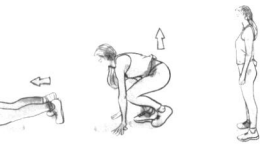

SET 1 REPS: _____   →   15s REST
SET 2 REPS: _____   →   15s REST
SET 3 REPS: _____   →   15s REST
SET 4 REPS: _____   →   15s REST

--- 30 SECOND BREAK ---

COOL DOWN
60s EACH

a. Hamstring Stretch **b. Glute Stretch** **c. Pigeon Stretch** **d. Runner's Stretch**

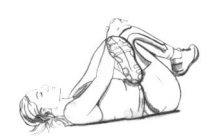

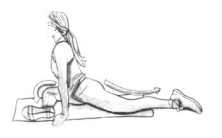

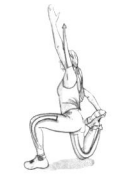

TODAY'S WORKOUT INTENSITY: _____ / 10

EXERCISE GUIDE
https://HabitNest.link/booty02

Workout 2: 4-3-2-1

DATE _____

GLUTE ACTIVATION WARMUP
30s EACH

a. Clam Opener

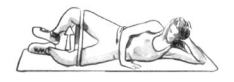

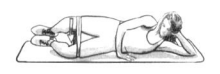

b. Lateral Leg Raise

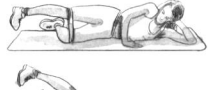

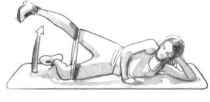

c. Glute Bridge w/ Leg Extension

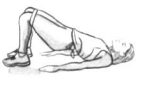

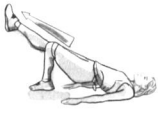

d. Tabletop w/ Diagonal Kick

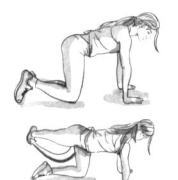

(30s Each Side)

- 30s Each Leg (w/ Foot Flexed)
- 30s Each Leg (w/ Toes Pointing Down)

(30s Each Leg)

(30s Each Leg)

--- 30 SECOND BREAK ---

CIRCUIT 1
60s EACH

1a. Burpee

1b. Reverse Dumbbell Fly

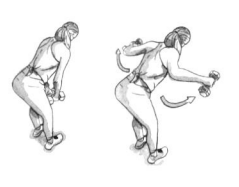

1c. Mountain Climber

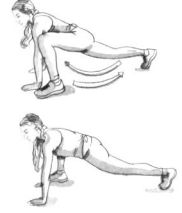

1d. Starfish Crunch

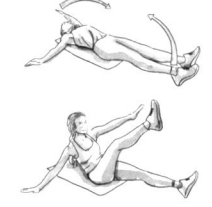

REPS: _____ → REPS: _____ → REPS: _____ → REPS: _____
(Alternate Sides)　(Alternate Sides)

--- 30 SECOND BREAK ---

CIRCUIT 2
50s EACH

2a. Jump Twist

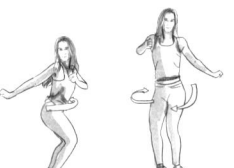

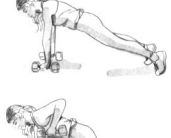

2b. Plank to Row

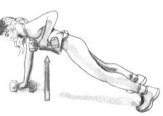

2c. Vertical Sit-Up w/ Elbow to Knee Touch

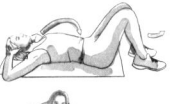

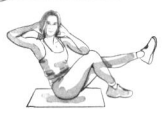

SET 1 REPS: _____ → SET 1 REPS: _____ → SET 1 REPS: _____
(Alternate Sides)　(Alternate Sides)

SET 2 REPS: _____ → SET 2 REPS: _____ → SET 2 REPS: _____
(Alternate Sides)　(Alternate Sides)

―――― 30 SECOND BREAK ――――

CIRCUIT 3
40s EACH

(Feel free to substitute any one exercise out for another that you feel will fit your goals / needs better! Make this journal your own!)

3a. Side Plank w/ Elbow Twist

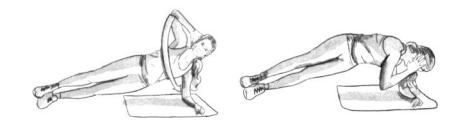

3b. Fast Feet

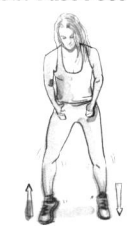

(Left Side)   SET 1 REPS: _____ → SET 1 REPS: _____

(Right Side)   SET 2 REPS: _____ → SET 2 REPS: _____

(Alternate Sides)   SET 3 REPS: _____ → SET 3 REPS: _____

―――― 30 SECOND BREAK ――――

CIRCUIT 4
30s EACH

4a. Squat to Overhead Press

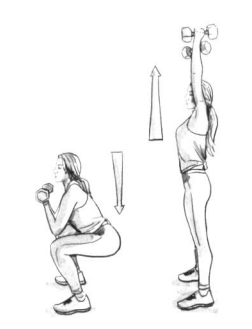

SET 1 REPS: _____ → 15s REST

SET 2 REPS: _____ → 15s REST

SET 3 REPS: _____ → 15s REST

SET 4 REPS: _____ → 15s REST

―――― 30 SECOND BREAK ――――

COOL DOWN
60s EACH

a. Runner's Stretch   **b. Butterfly Stretch**   **c. Lat Stretch**   **d. Crossbody Hangover**

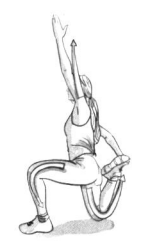

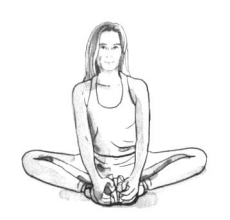

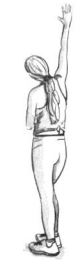

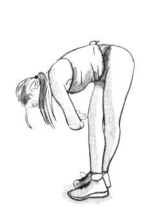

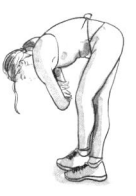

TODAY'S WORKOUT INTENSITY: _____ / 10

A quick note from our team:

<u>Happy with your journal so far?</u>

We worked very hard to build this - it would mean the absolute WORLD if you could share an honest review of your experience with it wherever you purchased your journal from.

<u>Having any issues or problems?</u>

This is one of our early runs of this journal - we know we have ways to improve it, so if you're having anything less than a 5-star experience PLEASE email us at support@habitnest.com so we can learn how to improve / see what we can do for you.

Regardless, we won't rest until you have an incredible experience here... promise :)

With love,
Jennifer, Ari, Amir, & Mikey

Workout 3: Resistance Training

DATE _____

1. Deadlift

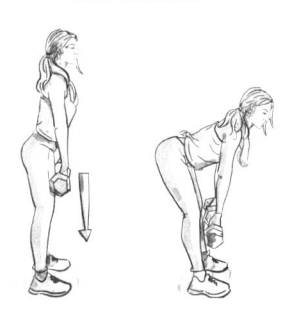

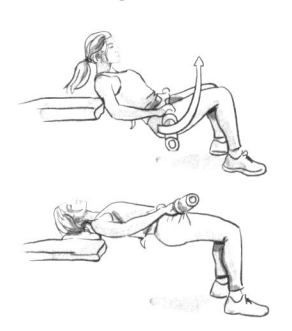

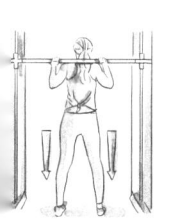

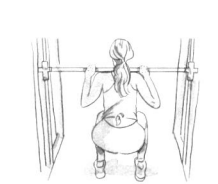

SET 1 REPS: _____ (GOAL: 15-20) WEIGHT: _____

SET 2 REPS: _____ (GOAL: 12-15) WEIGHT: _____

SET 3 REPS: _____ (GOAL: 10-12) WEIGHT: _____

SET 4 REPS: _____ (GOAL: 8-10) WEIGHT: _____
(Optional)

(Life hack: If you use this journal's elastic band to hold it closed, the band doubles up as a pen holder. Slide your pen clip through it, allowing your pen to rest on top of the book!)

2. Hip Thrust

SET 1 REPS: _____ (GOAL: 15-20) WEIGHT: _____

SET 2 REPS: _____ (GOAL: 12-15) WEIGHT: _____

SET 3 REPS: _____ (GOAL: 10-12) WEIGHT: _____

SET 4 REPS: _____ (GOAL: 8-10) WEIGHT: _____
(Optional)

(Note: You can do all these exercises without equipment at home if you'd like.)

3. Squat

SET 1 REPS: _____ (GOAL: 15-20) WEIGHT: _____

SET 2 REPS: _____ (GOAL: 12-15) WEIGHT: _____

SET 3 REPS: _____ (GOAL: 10-12) WEIGHT: _____

SET 4 REPS: _____ (GOAL: 8-10) WEIGHT: _____
(Optional)

4. Alternating Step Up

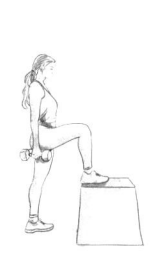

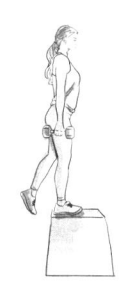

SET 1 REPS: _____ (GOAL: 15-20) WEIGHT: _____

SET 2 REPS: _____ (GOAL: 12-15) WEIGHT: _____

SET 3 REPS: _____ (GOAL: 10-12) WEIGHT: _____

SET 4 REPS: _____ (GOAL: 8-10) WEIGHT: _____
(Optional)

TODAY'S WORKOUT INTENSITY: _____ / 10

EXERCISE GUIDE
https://HabitNest.link/booty03

Workout 4: 4-3-2-1

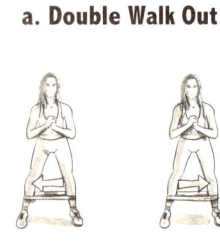

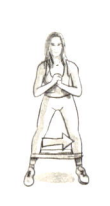

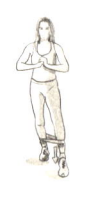

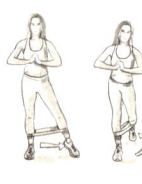

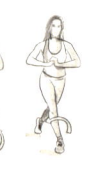

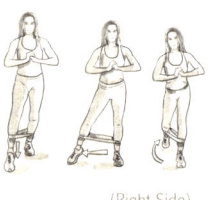

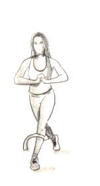

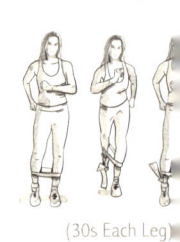

EXERCISE GUIDE
https://HabitNest.link/booty04

DATE _____

GLUTE ACTIVATION WARMUP
(30s EACH)

a. Double Walk Out
(2 Steps Right, 2 Steps Left)

b. Box Draw
(Left Side)

c. Box Draw
(Right Side)

d. Running M...
(30s Each Leg)

(Note: If using a glute band is too difficult, feel free to do these warmups without one.)

--- 30 SECOND BREAK ---

CIRCUIT 1
(60s EACH)

1a. Burpee

1b. Bulgarian Lunge

1c. Bulgarian Lunge

1d. Mountain Clim...

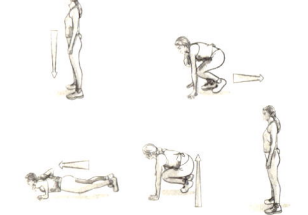

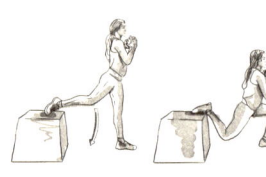

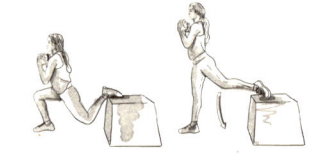

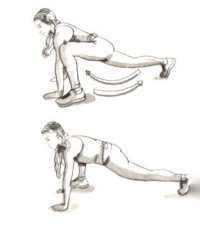

REPS: _____ → REPS: _____ (Right Leg) → REPS: _____ (Left Leg) → REPS: _____ (Alternate Sides)

--- 30 SECOND BREAK ---

CIRCUIT 2
(50s EACH)

2a. Jump Lunge

2b. Single Leg Glute Bridge

2c. Speed Skater

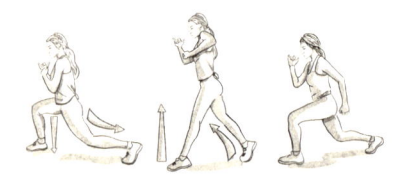

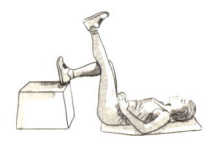

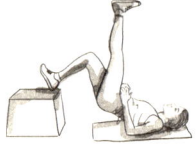

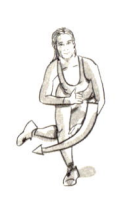

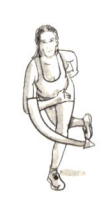

SET 1 REPS: _____ (Alternate Legs) → SET 1 REPS: _____ (Left Leg) → SET 1 REPS: _____ (Alternate Sides)

SET 2 REPS: _____ (Alternate Legs) → SET 2 REPS: _____ (Right Leg) → SET 2 REPS: _____ (Alternate Sides)

--- 30 SECOND BREAK ---

CIRCUIT 3
40s EACH

3a. Russian Twist

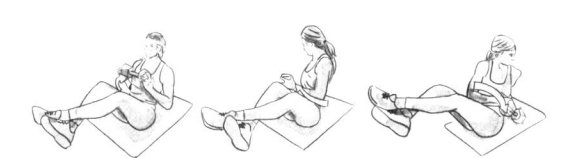

3b. Side Shuffle w/ Floor Tap

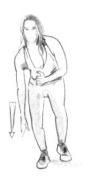

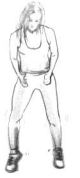

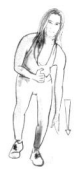

(Left Side)   SET 1 REPS: _____ →   SET 1 REPS: _____

(Right Side)   SET 2 REPS: _____ →   SET 2 REPS: _____

(Alternate Sides)   SET 3 REPS: _____ →   SET 3 REPS: _____

--- 30 SECOND BREAK ---

CIRCUIT 4
30s EACH

4a. Squat Jack

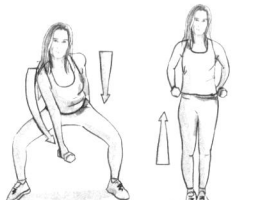

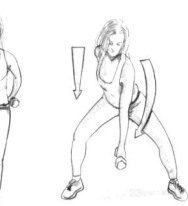

SET 1 REPS: _____ → 15s REST

SET 2 REPS: _____ → 15s REST

SET 3 REPS: _____ → 15s REST

SET 4 REPS: _____ → 15s REST

--- 30 SECOND BREAK ---

COOL DOWN
60s EACH

a. Hamstring Stretch

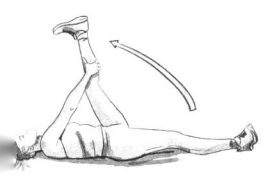

b. Pigeon Stretch

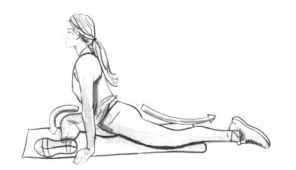

c. Glute Stretch

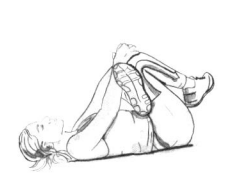

d. Lat Stretch

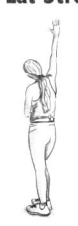

TODAY'S WORKOUT INTENSITY: _____ / 10

Psssstt... We like rewarding people (like you) who TAKE ACTION and actually use this journal.

Email us now at secret+booty@habitnest.com for a secret gift ;)

Workout 5: Resistance Training

DATE _____

1. Shoulder Rope Pull

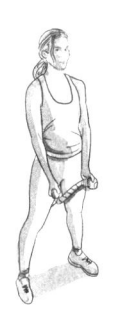

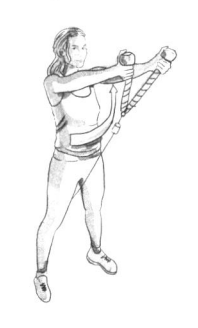

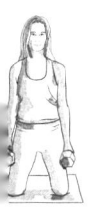

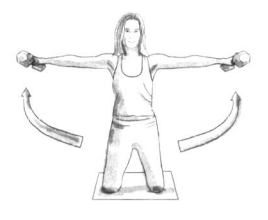

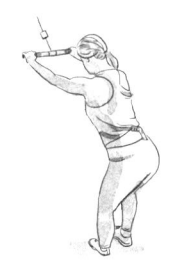

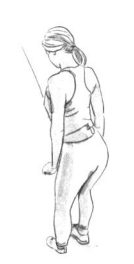

SET 1 REPS: _____ (GOAL: 15-20) WEIGHT: _____
SET 2 REPS: _____ (GOAL: 12-15) WEIGHT: _____
SET 3 REPS: _____ (GOAL: 10-12) WEIGHT: _____
SET 4 REPS: _____ (GOAL: 8-10)   WEIGHT: _____
(Optional)

2. Lateral Raise

SET 1 REPS: _____ (GOAL: 15-20) WEIGHT: _____
SET 2 REPS: _____ (GOAL: 12-15) WEIGHT: _____
SET 3 REPS: _____ (GOAL: 10-12) WEIGHT: _____
SET 4 REPS: _____ (GOAL: 8-10)   WEIGHT: _____
(Optional)

3. Straight Arm Rope Pull

SET 1 REPS: _____ (GOAL: 15-20) WEIGHT: _____
SET 2 REPS: _____ (GOAL: 12-15) WEIGHT: _____
SET 3 REPS: _____ (GOAL: 10-12) WEIGHT: _____
SET 4 REPS: _____ (GOAL: 8-10)   WEIGHT: _____
(Optional)

4. Cable Row w/Squat

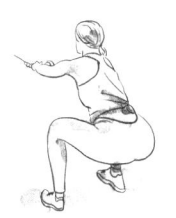

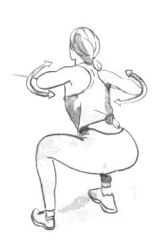

SET 1 REPS: _____ (GOAL: 15-20) WEIGHT: _____
SET 2 REPS: _____ (GOAL: 12-15) WEIGHT: _____
SET 3 REPS: _____ (GOAL: 10-12) WEIGHT: _____
SET 4 REPS: _____ (GOAL: 8-10)   WEIGHT: _____
(Optional)

TODAY'S WORKOUT INTENSITY: _____ / 10

EXERCISE GUIDE
https://HabitNest.link/booty05

EXERCISE GUIDE
https://HabitNest.link/booty06

Workout 6: 4-3-2-1

DATE _____

GLUTE ACTIVATION WARMUP (30s EACH)

a. Double Walk Out
(2 Steps Right, 2 Steps Left)

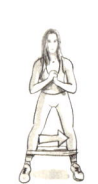

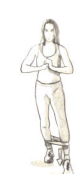

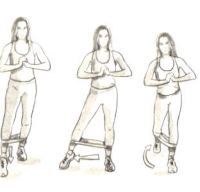

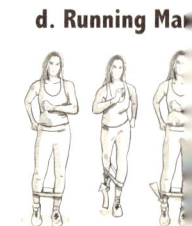

b. Box Draw
(Left Side)

c. Box Draw
(Right Side)

d. Running Ma[n]
(30s Each Leg)

---- 30 SECOND BREAK ----

CIRCUIT 1 (60s EACH)

1a. Vertical Leap
REPS: _____ →

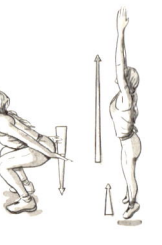

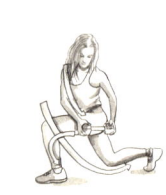

1b. Woodchopper
REPS: _____
(Right Side) →

1b. Woodchopper
REPS: _____
(Left Side) →

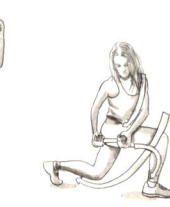

1d. The Heisman
REPS: _____

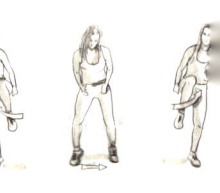

---- 30 SECOND BREAK ----

CIRCUIT 2 (50s EACH)

2a. Squat Thrust
SET 1 REPS: _____ →
SET 2 REPS: _____ →

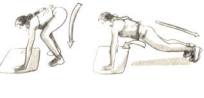

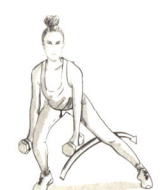

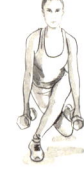

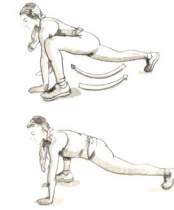

2b. Lateral Lunge to Curtsy Lunge
SET 1 REPS: _____
(Left Leg) →
SET 2 REPS: _____
(Right Leg) →

2c. Mountain Climber
SET 1 REPS: _____
(Alternate Sides)
SET 2 REPS: _____
(Alternate Sides)

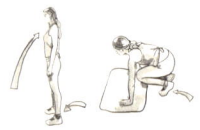

― 30 SECOND BREAK ―

CIRCUIT 3
(40s EACH)

3a. Lateral Lunge w/ Half 'X'

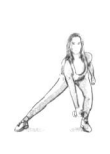

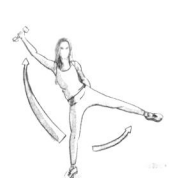

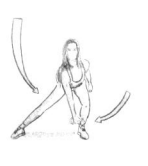

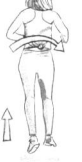

3b. 180° Jump Twist to Floor Tap

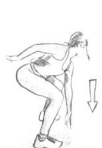

(Left Side)   SET 1 REPS: _____   →   SET 1 REPS: _____

(Right Side)   SET 2 REPS: _____   →   SET 2 REPS: _____

(Alternate Sides) SET 3 REPS: _____   →   SET 3 REPS: _____

― 30 SECOND BREAK ―

CIRCUIT 4
(30s EACH)

4a. Leap Forward in Squat, Burpee, & Shuffle Back

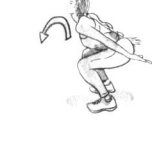

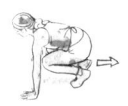

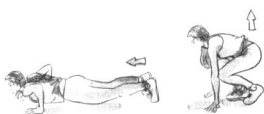

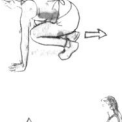

SET 1 REPS: _____   →   15s REST

SET 2 REPS: _____   →   15s REST

SET 3 REPS: _____   →   15s REST

SET 4 REPS: _____   →   15s REST

― 30 SECOND BREAK ―

COOL DOWN
(60s EACH)

a. Hamstring Stretch   **b. Crossbody Hangover**   **c. Runner's Stretch**   **d. Butterfly Stretch**

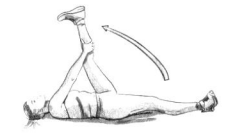

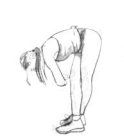

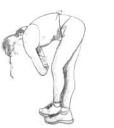

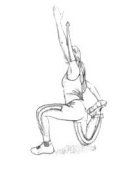

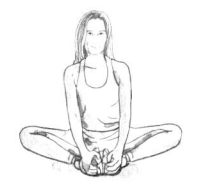

TODAY'S WORKOUT INTENSITY: _____ / 10

EXERCISE GUIDE
https://HabitNest.link/booty07

Workout 7: 4-3-2-1

DATE _____

GLUTE ACTIVATION WARMUP
30s EACH

a. Clam Opener

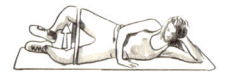

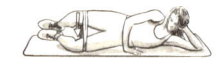

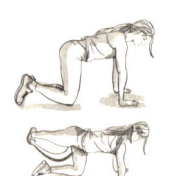

b. Tabletop w/ Diagonal Kick

c. Glute Bridge w/ Leg Extension

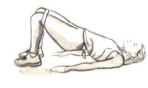

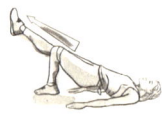

d. Fire Hydrant

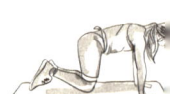

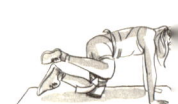

(30s Each Side) (30s Each Leg) (30s Each Leg) (30s Each Leg)

--- 30 SECOND BREAK ---

CIRCUIT 1
60s EACH

1a. Jump Twist   **1b. Side Triangle Crunch**   **1c. Side Triangle Crunch**   **1d. Reverse Dumbbell Fly**

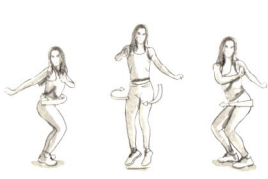

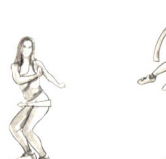

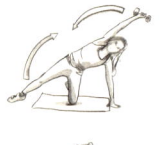

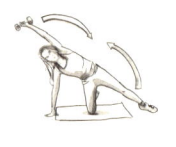

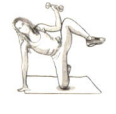

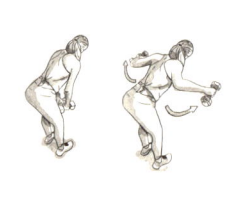

REPS: _____ → REPS: _____ → REPS: _____ → REPS: _____
                    (Right Side)   (Left Side)

--- 30 SECOND BREAK ---

CIRCUIT 2
50s EACH

2a. Speed Skater   **2b. Plank to Row**   **2c. V-Up**

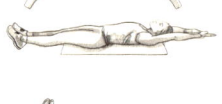

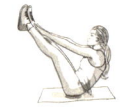

SET 1 REPS: _____ → SET 1 REPS: _____ → SET 1 REPS: _____
                          (Alternate Arms)

SET 2 REPS: _____ → SET 2 REPS: _____ → SET 2 REPS: _____
                          (Alternate Arms)

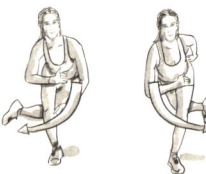

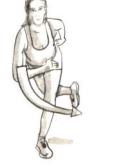

―― 30 SECOND BREAK ――

CIRCUIT 3
40s EACH

3a. Spider-Man Plank Crunch

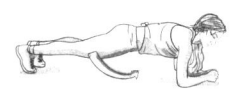

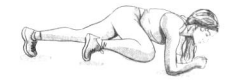

3b. Burpee

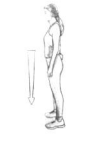

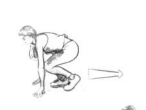

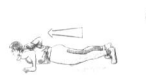

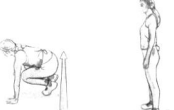

(Alternate Sides) SET 1 REPS: _____ → SET 1 REPS: _____
(Alternate Sides) SET 2 REPS: _____ → SET 2 REPS: _____
(Alternate Sides) SET 3 REPS: _____ → SET 3 REPS: _____

―― 30 SECOND BREAK ――

CIRCUIT 4
30s EACH

4a. Ski Mogul

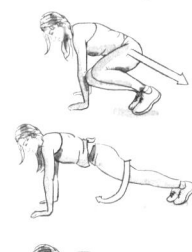

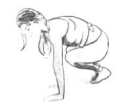

SET 1 REPS: _____ → 15s REST
SET 2 REPS: _____ → 15s REST
SET 3 REPS: _____ → 15s REST
SET 4 REPS: _____ → 15s REST

―― 30 SECOND BREAK ――

COOL DOWN
60s EACH

a. Glute Stretch　　**b. Butterfly Stretch**　　**c. Pigeon Stretch**　　**d. Lat Stretch**

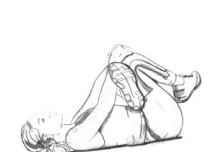

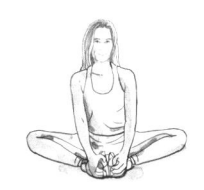

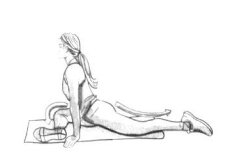

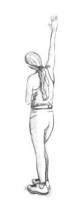

TODAY'S WORKOUT INTENSITY: _____ / 10

Workout 8: Resistance Training

DATE _____

1. Elevated Plie Squat

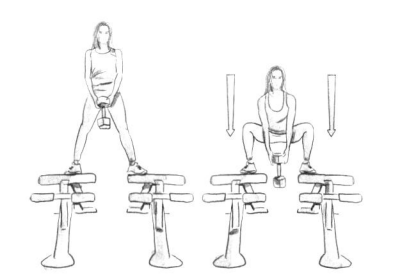

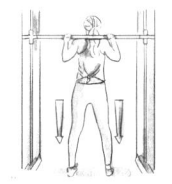

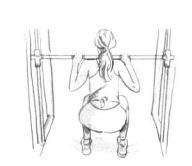

SET 1	REPS: _____	(GOAL: 15-20)	WEIGHT: _____
SET 2	REPS: _____	(GOAL: 12-15)	WEIGHT: _____
SET 3	REPS: _____	(GOAL: 10-12)	WEIGHT: _____
SET 4 (Optional)	REPS: _____	(GOAL: 8-10)	WEIGHT: _____

2. Woodchopper

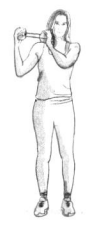

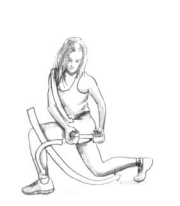

Left | Right

SET 1	REPS: _____	(GOAL: 15-20)	WEIGHT: _____
SET 2	REPS: _____	(GOAL: 12-15)	WEIGHT: _____
SET 3	REPS: _____	(GOAL: 10-12)	WEIGHT: _____
SET 4 (Optional)	REPS: _____	(GOAL: 8-10)	WEIGHT: _____

3. Squat

SET 1	REPS: _____	(GOAL: 15-20)	WEIGHT: _____
SET 2	REPS: _____	(GOAL: 12-15)	WEIGHT: _____
SET 3	REPS: _____	(GOAL: 10-12)	WEIGHT: _____
SET 4 (Optional)	REPS: _____	(GOAL: 8-10)	WEIGHT: _____

4. Hip Thrust

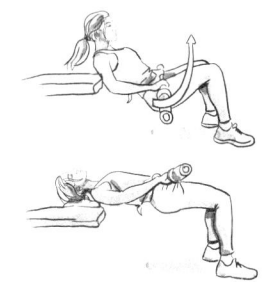

SET 1	REPS: _____	(GOAL: 15-20)	WEIGHT: _____
SET 2	REPS: _____	(GOAL: 12-15)	WEIGHT: _____
SET 3	REPS: _____	(GOAL: 10-12)	WEIGHT: _____
SET 4 (Optional)	REPS: _____	(GOAL: 8-10)	WEIGHT: _____

EXERCISE GUIDE
https://HabitNest.link/booty08

TODAY'S WORKOUT INTENSITY: _____ / 10

EXERCISE GUIDE
https://HabitNest.link/booty09

Workout 9: 4-3-2-1

DATE

GLUTE ACTIVATION WARMUP
30s EACH

a. Double Walk Out
(2 Steps Right, 2 Steps Left)

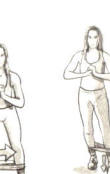

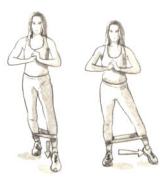

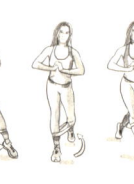

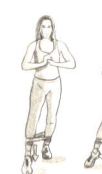

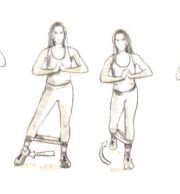

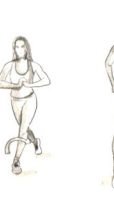

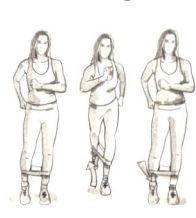

b. Box Draw
(Left Side)

c. Box Draw
(Right Side)

d. Running Man
(30s Each Leg)

--- 30 SECOND BREAK ---

CIRCUIT 1
60s EACH

1a. High Knee
REPS: _____

1b. Bulgarian Lunge
REPS: _____
(Right Leg)

1c. Bulgarian Lunge
REPS: _____
(Left Leg)

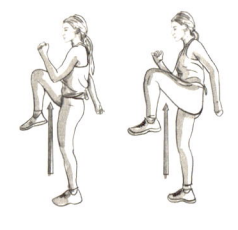

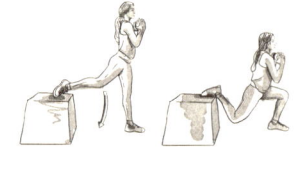

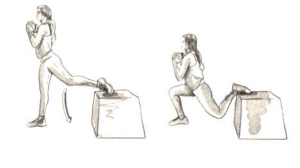

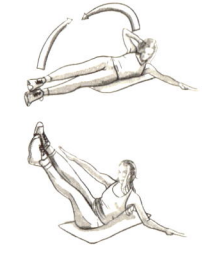

1d. Side V-Up
REPS: _____
(30s Each Side)

--- 30 SECOND BREAK ---

CIRCUIT 2
50s EACH

2a. Side Shuffle w/ Floor Tap
SET 1 REPS: _____
SET 2 REPS: _____

2b. Plank Step Up
SET 1 REPS: _____
SET 2 REPS: _____

2c. In and Out Jack
SET 1 REPS: _____
SET 2 REPS: _____

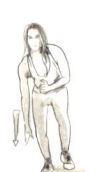

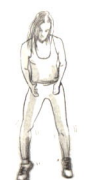

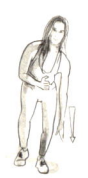

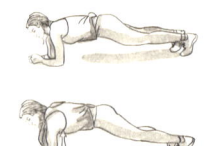

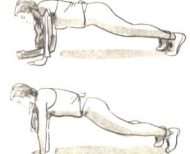

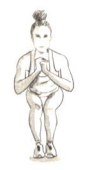

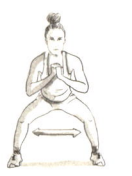

--- 30 SECOND BREAK ---

CIRCUIT 3
40s EACH

3a. Side Plank w/ Torso Twist

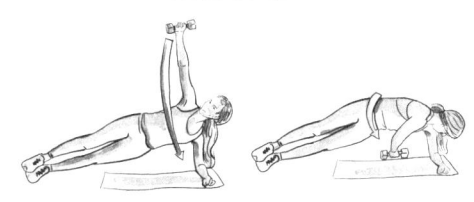

3b. Lateral Lunge w/ Half 'X'

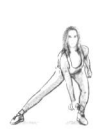

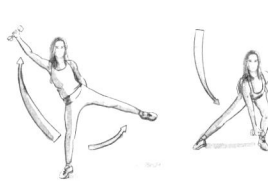

(Left Side)   SET 1 REPS: _____ → (Left Side)   SET 1 REPS: _____

(Right Side)   SET 2 REPS: _____ → (Right Side)   SET 2 REPS: _____

(Alternate Side)   SET 3 REPS: _____ → (Alternate Side)   SET 3 REPS: _____

--- 30 SECOND BREAK ---

CIRCUIT 4
30s EACH

4a. Pendulum Jack

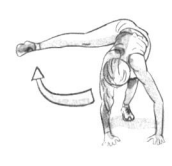

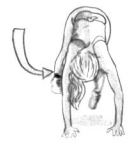

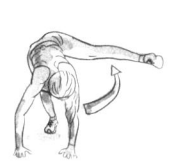

SET 1 REPS: _____ → 15s REST

SET 2 REPS: _____ → 15s REST

SET 3 REPS: _____ → 15s REST

SET 4 REPS: _____ → 15s REST

--- 30 SECOND BREAK ---

COOL DOWN
60s EACH

a. Hamstring Stretch　　**b. Runner's Stretch**　　**c. Butterfly Stretch**　　**d. Lat Stretch**

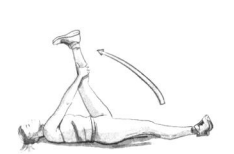

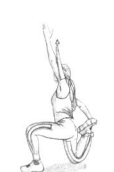

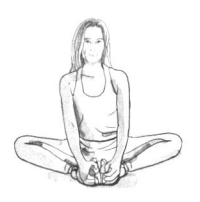

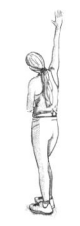

TODAY'S WORKOUT INTENSITY: _____ / 10

Workout 10: Resistance Training

DATE _____

1. Reverse Dumbbell Fly

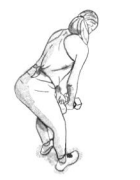

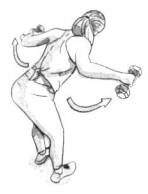

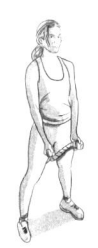

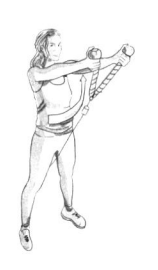

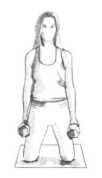

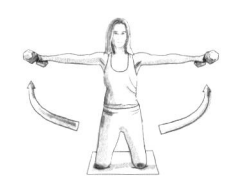

SET 1	REPS: _____	(GOAL: 15-20)	WEIGHT: _____
SET 2	REPS: _____	(GOAL: 12-15)	WEIGHT: _____
SET 3	REPS: _____	(GOAL: 10-12)	WEIGHT: _____
SET 4 (Optional)	REPS: _____	(GOAL: 8-10)	WEIGHT: _____

2. Shoulder Rope Pull

SET 1	REPS: _____	(GOAL: 15-20)	WEIGHT: _____
SET 2	REPS: _____	(GOAL: 12-15)	WEIGHT: _____
SET 3	REPS: _____	(GOAL: 10-12)	WEIGHT: _____
SET 4 (Optional)	REPS: _____	(GOAL: 8-10)	WEIGHT: _____

3. Lateral Raise

SET 1	REPS: _____	(GOAL: 15-20)	WEIGHT: _____
SET 2	REPS: _____	(GOAL: 12-15)	WEIGHT: _____
SET 3	REPS: _____	(GOAL: 10-12)	WEIGHT: _____
SET 4 (Optional)	REPS: _____	(GOAL: 8-10)	WEIGHT: _____

4. Arnold Press

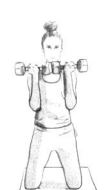

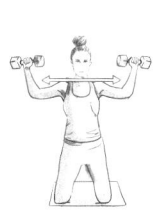

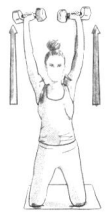

SET 1	REPS: _____	(GOAL: 15-20)	WEIGHT: _____
SET 2	REPS: _____	(GOAL: 12-15)	WEIGHT: _____
SET 3	REPS: _____	(GOAL: 10-12)	WEIGHT: _____
SET 4 (Optional)	REPS: _____	(GOAL: 8-10)	WEIGHT: _____

EXERCISE GUIDE
https://HabitNest.link/booty10

TODAY'S WORKOUT INTENSITY: _____ / 10

Check-In

Taking a few minutes to simply STOP and evaluate how you're doing mentally, physically, and emotionally every few weeks of a training program can be extremely helpful to your experience with the program.

Take a few minutes to answer the following questions with honesty!

What is my goal in completing this process - how do I want to look, feel, and what do I expect from doing this?

_____
_____
_____
_____

How am I feeling about the quality and intensity of my workouts? Can I do more or am I pushing the limit consistently? Am I getting enough rest?

_____
_____
_____
_____

How is my new workout routine benefitting my mindset?

_____
_____
_____
_____

What do I want to learn about this process that I can spend some time researching?

_____
_____
_____
_____

Pro-Tip

> *The Importance of Resistance Training for Health*

As we age, resistance training becomes increasingly important.

Around the age of 30, we start losing muscle mass and function more quickly. There's actually a medical term for this - *Sarcopenia*.

This happens even in people who stay physically active but aren't necessarily strength training.

There is a reduction in the nerve cells responsible for sending signals from the brain to our muscles for movement.

Our ability to turn protein into energy lessens. Our risk of injury increases and our bones are less protected.

Strength training not only comes with all the psychological benefits of increased well-being and self-esteem, but a wide host of physical health benefits.

It protects our bones, prevents becoming frail as we age, protects our joints, increases our stamina for everyday life, improves posture, mobility and balance, improves sleep, and actually enhances our performance of everyday tasks.

Strength training and proper muscle development are critically important to living a long, healthy life. They should be a part of all of our lives in some way or another.

And it's never too late or too early to start!

EXERCISE GUIDE
https://HabitNest.link/booty11

Workout 11: 4-3-2-1

DATE _____

GLUTE ACTIVATION WARMUP
(30s Each)

a. Clam Opener

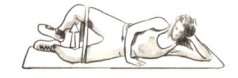

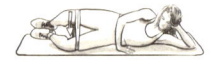

b. Glute Bridge w/ Band Flutter

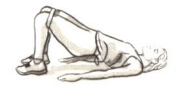

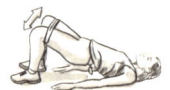

c. Fire Hydrant

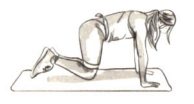

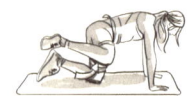

d. Lateral Leg Raise

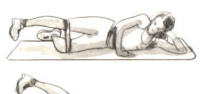

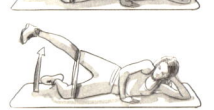

(30s Each Side)

(30s Each Side)

- 30s Each Leg (w/ Foot Flexed)
- 30s Each Leg (w/ Toes Pointing Down)

--- 30 SECOND BREAK ---

CIRCUIT 1
(60s Each)

1a. Vertical Leap

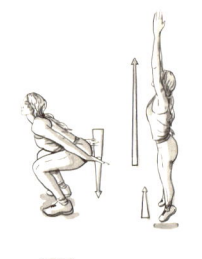

1b. Lateral Lunge to Curtsy Lunge

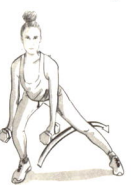

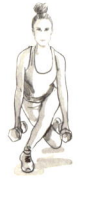

1c. Lateral Lunge to Curtsy Lunge

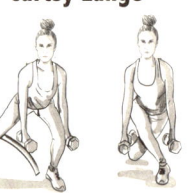

1d. Squat Thrust

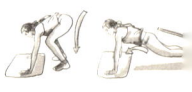

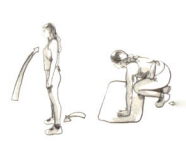

REPS: _____ → REPS: _____ (Right Side) → REPS: _____ (Left Side) → REPS: _____

--- 30 SECOND BREAK ---

CIRCUIT 2
(50s Each)

2a. Russian Twist

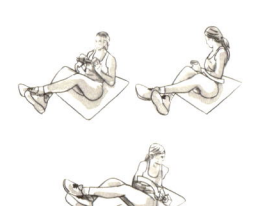

2b. Plie Jump Squat

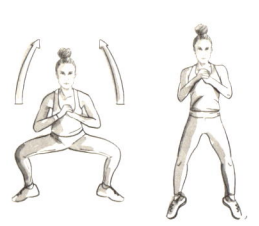

2c. Ski Mogul

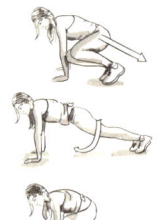

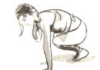

SET 1 REPS: _____ → SET 1 REPS: _____ → SET 1 REPS: _____

SET 2 REPS: _____ → SET 2 REPS: _____ → SET 2 REPS: _____

─── 30 SECOND BREAK ───

CIRCUIT 3
40s EACH

3a. Roundhouse Kick to Squat

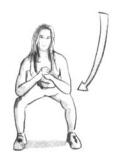

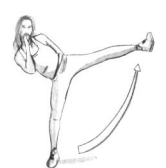

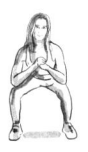

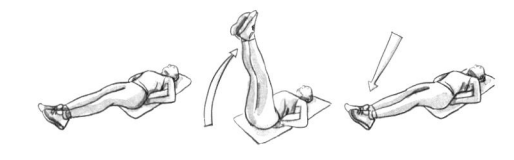

3b. Leg Drop

(Left Leg)   SET 1 REPS: _____   →   SET 1 REPS: _____
(Right Leg)   SET 2 REPS: _____   →   SET 2 REPS: _____
(Alternate Legs) SET 3 REPS: _____   →   SET 3 REPS: _____

─── 30 SECOND BREAK ───

CIRCUIT 4
30s EACH

4a. Burpee

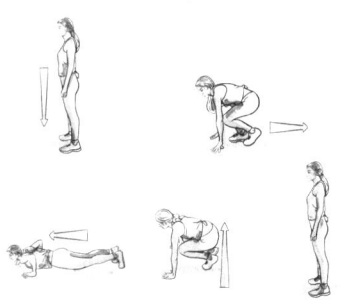

SET 1 REPS: _____   →   15s REST
SET 2 REPS: _____   →   15s REST
SET 3 REPS: _____   →   15s REST
SET 4 REPS: _____   →   15s REST

─── 30 SECOND BREAK ───

COOL DOWN
60s EACH

a. Hamstring Stretch   **b. Pigeon Stretch**   **c. Lat Stretch**   **d. Butterfly Stretch**

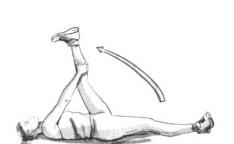

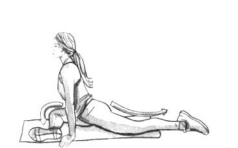

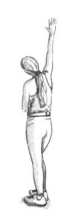

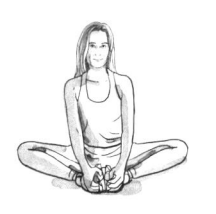

TODAY'S WORKOUT INTENSITY: _____ / 10

EXERCISE GUIDE
https://HabitNest.link/booty12

Workout 12: 4-3-2-1

DATE _____

GLUTE ACTIVATION WARMUP
(30s EACH)

a. Clam Opener

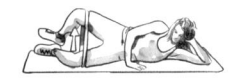

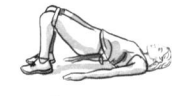

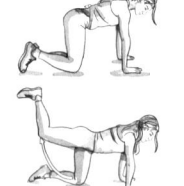

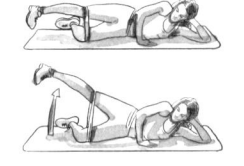

(30s Each Side)

b. Glute Bridge w/ Band Flutter

c. Tabletop w/Donkey Kick

d. Lateral Leg Raise

- 30s Each Leg (w/ Foot Flexed)
- 30s Each Leg (w/ Toes Pointing Down)

--- 30 SECOND BREAK ---

CIRCUIT 1
(60s EACH)

1a. Mountain Climber

REPS: _____ →

1b. Side V-Up

REPS: _____
(Right Side) →

1c. Side V-Up

REPS: _____
(Left Side) →

1d. High Knee

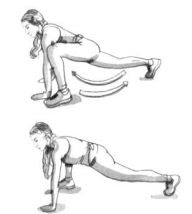

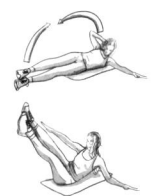

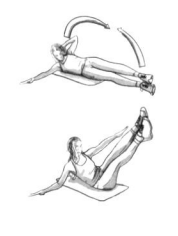

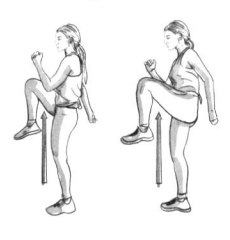

REPS: _____

--- 30 SECOND BREAK ---

CIRCUIT 2
(50s EACH)

2a. Starfish Crunch

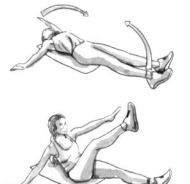

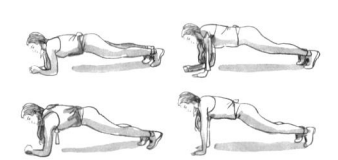

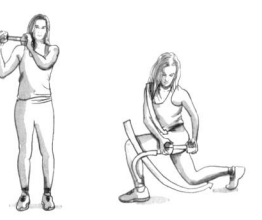

SET 1 REPS: _____
(Alternate Arms) →

SET 2 REPS: _____
(Alternate Arms)

2b. Plank Step Up

SET 1 REPS: _____
(Alternate Arms) →

SET 2 REPS: _____
(Alternate Arms)

2c. Woodchopper

SET 1 REPS: _____
(Left Side)

SET 2 REPS: _____
(Right Side)

--- 30 SECOND BREAK ---

CIRCUIT 3
40s EACH

3a. Plie Squat w/ Shoulder Windmill

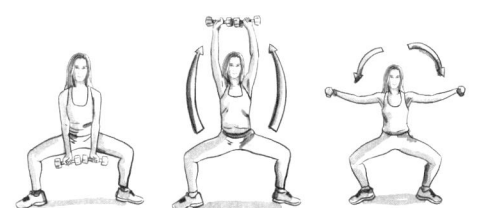

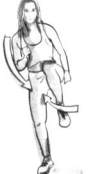

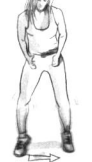

3b. The Heisman

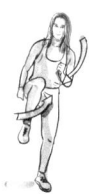

SET 1 REPS: _____ → SET 1 REPS: _____

SET 2 REPS: _____ → SET 2 REPS: _____

SET 3 REPS: _____ → SET 3 REPS: _____

--- 30 SECOND BREAK ---

CIRCUIT 4
30s EACH

4a. 180° Jump Twist to Floor Tap

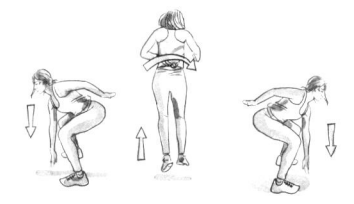

SET 1 REPS: _____ → 15s REST

SET 2 REPS: _____ → 15s REST

SET 3 REPS: _____ → 15s REST

SET 4 REPS: _____ → 15s REST

--- 30 SECOND BREAK ---

COOL DOWN
60s EACH

a. Pigeon Stretch   **b. Hamstring Stretch**   **c. Lat Stretch**   **d. Glute Stretch**

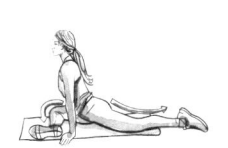

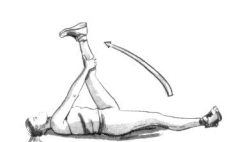

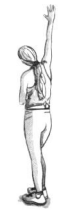

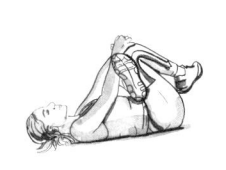

TODAY'S WORKOUT INTENSITY: _____ / 10

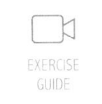

Workout 13: Resistance Training

DATE _____

https://HabitNest.link/booty13

1. Single Leg Deadlift

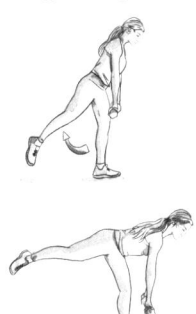

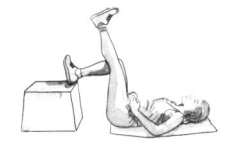

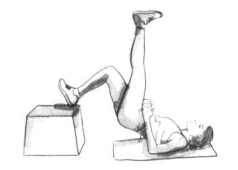

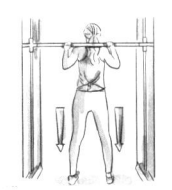

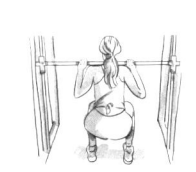

	Left	Right	
SET 1	REPS: _____	(GOAL: 15-20)	WEIGHT: _____
SET 2	REPS: _____	(GOAL: 12-15)	WEIGHT: _____
SET 3	REPS: _____	(GOAL: 10-12)	WEIGHT: _____
SET 4 (Optional)	REPS: _____	(GOAL: 8-10)	WEIGHT: _____

2. Single Leg Glute Bridge

	Left	Right	
SET 1	REPS: _____	(GOAL: 15-20)	WEIGHT: _____
SET 2	REPS: _____	(GOAL: 12-15)	WEIGHT: _____
SET 3	REPS: _____	(GOAL: 10-12)	WEIGHT: _____
SET 4 (Optional)	REPS: _____	(GOAL: 8-10)	WEIGHT: _____

3. Squat

SET 1 REPS: _____ (GOAL: 15-20) WEIGHT: _____
SET 2 REPS: _____ (GOAL: 12-15) WEIGHT: _____
SET 3 REPS: _____ (GOAL: 10-12) WEIGHT: _____
SET 4 (Optional) REPS: _____ (GOAL: 8-10) WEIGHT: _____

4. Hip Thrust

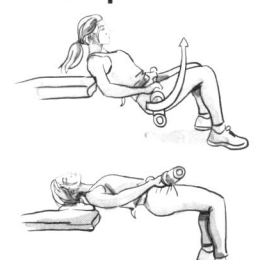

SET 1 REPS: _____ (GOAL: 15-20) WEIGHT: _____
SET 2 REPS: _____ (GOAL: 12-15) WEIGHT: _____
SET 3 REPS: _____ (GOAL: 10-12) WEIGHT: _____
SET 4 (Optional) REPS: _____ (GOAL: 8-10) WEIGHT: _____

TODAY'S WORKOUT INTENSITY: _____ / 10

Workout 14: 4-3-2-1

EXERCISE GUIDE
https://HabitNest.link/booty14

DATE: _____

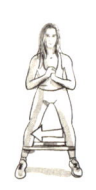

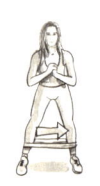

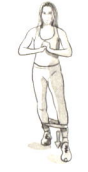

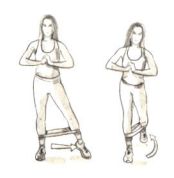

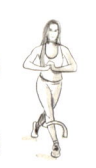

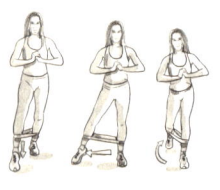

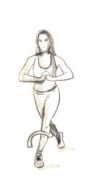

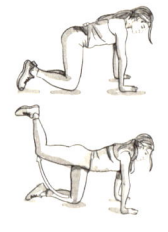

GLUTE ACTIVATION WARMUP
30s EACH

a. Double Walk Out
(2 Steps Right, 2 Steps Left)

b. Box Draw
(Left Side)

c. Box Draw
(Right Side)

d. Tabletop w/Donkey Kick
(30s Each Leg)

--- 30 SECOND BREAK ---

CIRCUIT 1
60s EACH

1a. Plie Jump Squat
REPS: _____

→

1b. Lateral Lunge w/ Half 'X'
REPS: _____
(Right Side)

→

1c. Lateral Lunge w/ Half 'X'
REPS: _____
(Left Side)

→

1d. Spider-Man Plank Crunch
REPS: _____
(Alternate Sides)

--- 30 SECOND BREAK ---

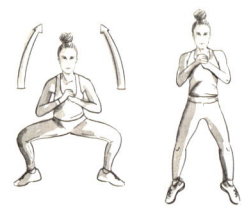

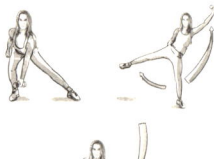

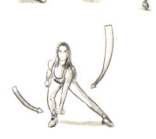

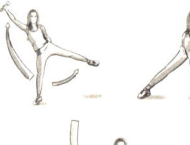

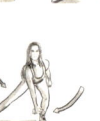

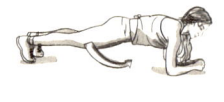

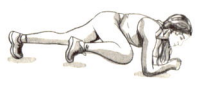

CIRCUIT 2
50s EACH

2a. Standing Side Crunch
SET 1 REPS: _____ (Left Side)
SET 2 REPS: _____ (Right Side)

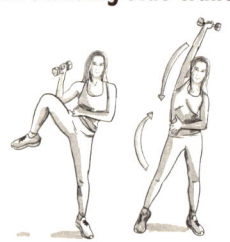

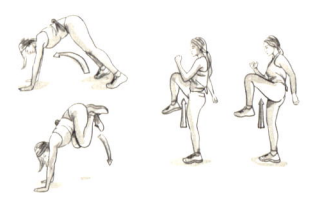

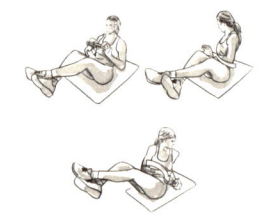

→

2b. 4 Donkey Kicks to 4 High Knees
SET 1 REPS: _____
SET 2 REPS: _____

→

2c. Russian Twist
SET 1 REPS: _____
SET 2 REPS: _____

---

30 SECOND BREAK

CIRCUIT 3
40s EACH

3a. 3-Point Lunge   ### 3b. In and Out Jack

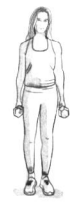

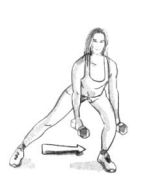

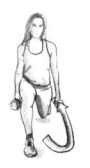

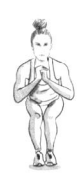

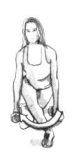

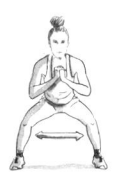

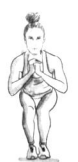

(Left Side)   SET 1 REPS: _____ → SET 1 REPS: _____

(Right Side)   SET 2 REPS: _____ → SET 2 REPS: _____

(Alternate Sides) SET 3 REPS: _____ → SET 3 REPS: _____

---

30 SECOND BREAK

CIRCUIT 4
30s EACH

4a. Burpee

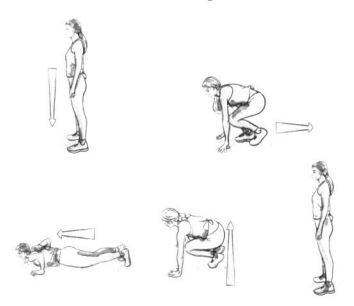

SET 1 REPS: _____ → 15s REST

SET 2 REPS: _____ → 15s REST

SET 3 REPS: _____ → 15s REST

SET 4 REPS: _____ → 15s REST

---

30 SECOND BREAK

COOL DOWN
60s EACH

a. Butterfly Stretch   **b. Runner's Stretch**   **c. Crossbody Hangover**   **d. Lat Stretch**

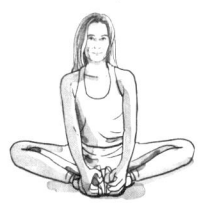

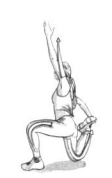

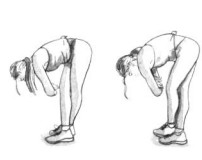

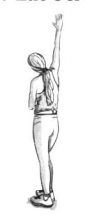

TODAY'S WORKOUT INTENSITY: _____ / 10

Note: We LOVE sharing stories of our users and what their lives looked like BEFORE using the journal compared to where they are NOW!

If you want to share your story with us, you can do so here:
habitnest.com/badasstestimonial

EXERCISE GUIDE
https://HabitNest.link/booty15

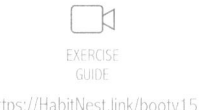

Workout 15: Resistance Training

DATE _____

1. Lateral Raise

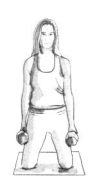

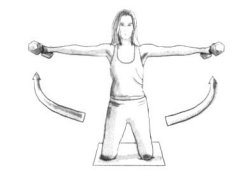

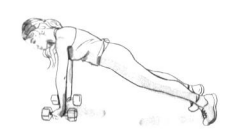

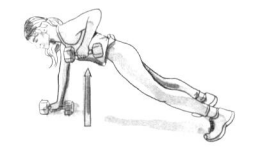

SET 1	REPS: _____ (GOAL: 15-20)	WEIGHT: _____
SET 2	REPS: _____ (GOAL: 12-15)	WEIGHT: _____
SET 3	REPS: _____ (GOAL: 10-12)	WEIGHT: _____
SET 4 (Optional)	REPS: _____ (GOAL: 8-10)	WEIGHT: _____

2. Shoulder Rope Pull

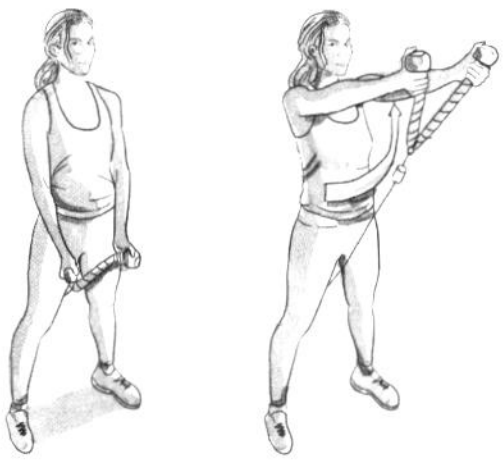

SET 1	REPS: _____ (GOAL: 15-20)	WEIGHT: _____
SET 2	REPS: _____ (GOAL: 12-15)	WEIGHT: _____
SET 3	REPS: _____ (GOAL: 10-12)	WEIGHT: _____
SET 4 (Optional)	REPS: _____ (GOAL: 8-10)	WEIGHT: _____

3. Plank to Row

SET 1	REPS: _____ (GOAL: 15-20)	WEIGHT: _____
SET 2	REPS: _____ (GOAL: 12-15)	WEIGHT: _____
SET 3	REPS: _____ (GOAL: 10-12)	WEIGHT: _____
SET 4 (Optional)	REPS: _____ (GOAL: 8-10)	WEIGHT: _____

4. Deadlift

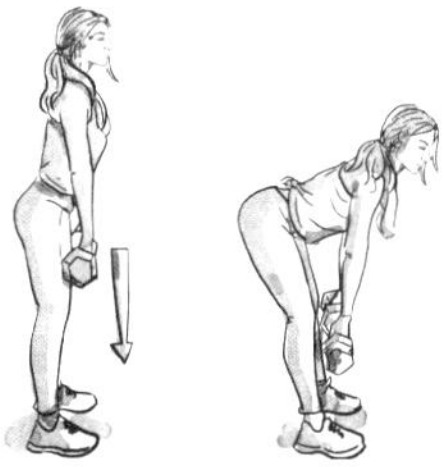

SET 1	REPS: _____ (GOAL: 15-20)	WEIGHT: _____
SET 2	REPS: _____ (GOAL: 12-15)	WEIGHT: _____
SET 3	REPS: _____ (GOAL: 10-12)	WEIGHT: _____
SET 4 (Optional)	REPS: _____ (GOAL: 8-10)	WEIGHT: _____

TODAY'S WORKOUT INTENSITY: _____ / 10

EXERCISE GUIDE
https://HabitNest.link/booty16

Workout 16: 4-3-2-1

DATE

GLUTE ACTIVATION WARMUP
30s EACH

a. Clam Opener

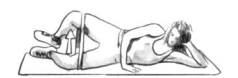

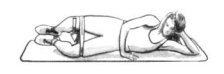

b. Glute Bridge w/ Band Flutter

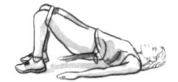

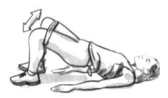

c. Fire Hydrant

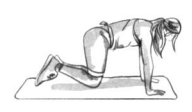

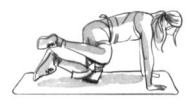

d. Double Walk Out

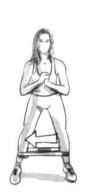

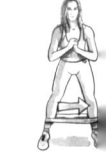

(30s Each Side)

(30s Each Leg)

(2 Steps Right, 2 Steps Left)

---30 SECOND BREAK---

CIRCUIT 1
60s EACH

1a. Ski Mogul

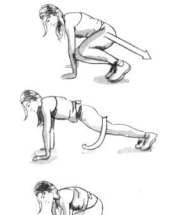

1b. Pendulum Lunge

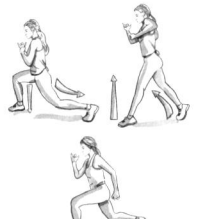

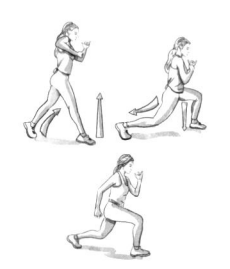

1c. Pendulum Lunge

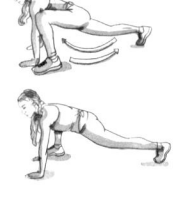

1d. Mountain Climber

REPS: _____ → REPS: _____ (Right Side) → REPS: _____ (Left Side) → REPS: _____ (Alternate Legs)

---30 SECOND BREAK---

CIRCUIT 2
50s EACH

2a. 3-Point Lunge

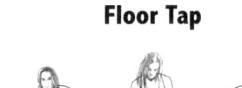

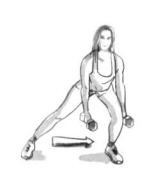

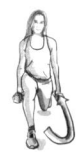

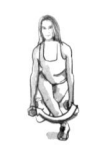

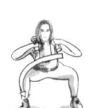

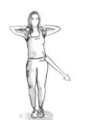

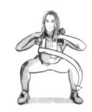

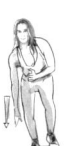

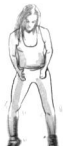

2b. Side to Side Squat

2c. Side Shuffle w/ Floor Tap

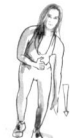

(Left Side) SET 1 REPS: _____ → SET 1 REPS: _____ → SET 1 REPS: _____

(Right Side) SET 2 REPS: _____ → SET 2 REPS: _____ → SET 2 REPS: _____

─── 30 SECOND BREAK ───

CIRCUIT 3
40s EACH

3a. Squat to Overhead Press

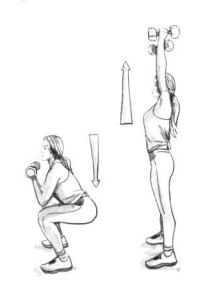

3b. Boxing Jab

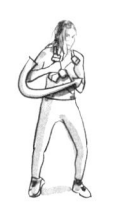

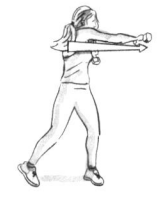

SET 1 REPS: _____ → SET 1 REPS: _____

SET 2 REPS: _____ → SET 2 REPS: _____

SET 3 REPS: _____ → SET 3 REPS: _____

─── 30 SECOND BREAK ───

CIRCUIT 4
30s EACH

4a. Jump Squat

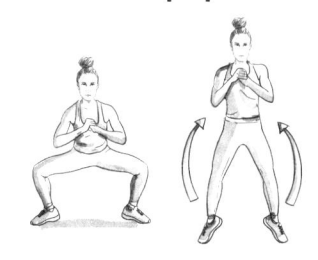

SET 1 REPS: _____ → 15s REST

SET 2 REPS: _____ → 15s REST

SET 3 REPS: _____ → 15s REST

SET 4 REPS: _____ → 15s REST

─── 30 SECOND BREAK ───

COOL DOWN
60s EACH

a. Pigeon Stretch   **b. Runner's Stretch**   **c. Crossbody Hangover**   **d. Hamstring Stretch**

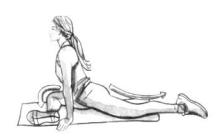

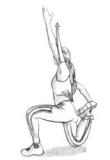

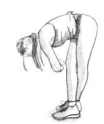

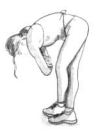

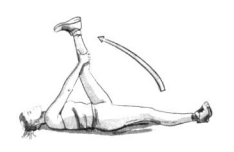

87

TODAY'S WORKOUT INTENSITY: _____ / 10

EXERCISE GUIDE
https://HabitNest.link/booty17

Workout 17: 4-3-2-1

DATE _____

GLUTE ACTIVATION WARMUP
(30s EACH)

a. Clam Opener

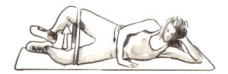

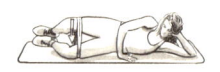

b. Glute Bridge w/ Band Flutter

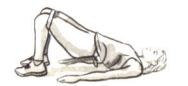

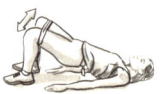

c. Fire Hydrant

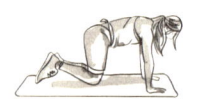

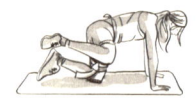

d. Lateral Leg Raise

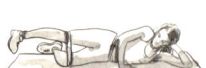

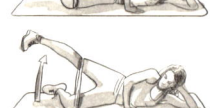

(30s Each Side)

(30s Each Side)

- 30s Each Leg (w/ Foot Flexed)
- 30s Each Leg (w/ Toes Pointing Down)

--- 30 SECOND BREAK ---

CIRCUIT 1
(60s EACH)

1a. In and Out Jack

1b. Leg Drop

1c. High Knee

1d. Russian Twist

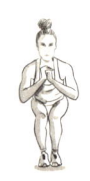

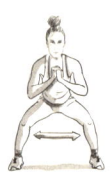

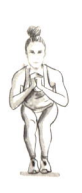

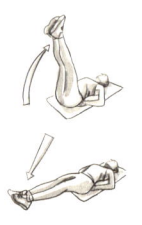

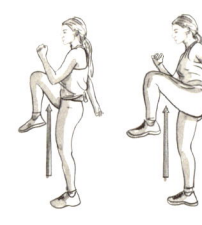

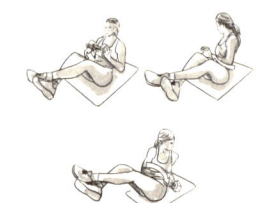

REPS: _____ → REPS: _____ → REPS: _____ → REPS: _____

--- 30 SECOND BREAK ---

CIRCUIT 2
(50s EACH)

2a. Plank Step Up

2b. Squat to Overhead Press

2c. Single Leg Glute Bridge

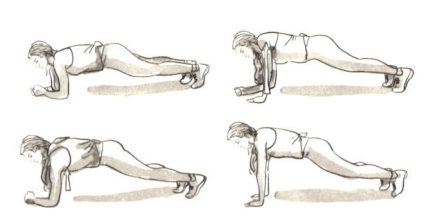

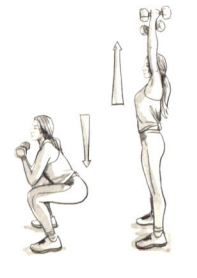

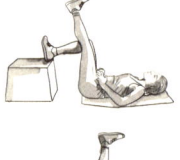

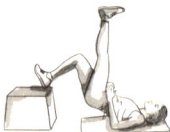

(Alternate Arms) SET 1 REPS: _____ → SET 1 REPS: _____ → (Left Leg) SET 1 REPS: _____

(Alternate Arms) SET 2 REPS: _____ → SET 2 REPS: _____ → (Right Leg) SET 2 REPS: _____

---

30 SECOND BREAK

CIRCUIT 3
(40s EACH)

3a. Side Plank w/ Torso Rotation

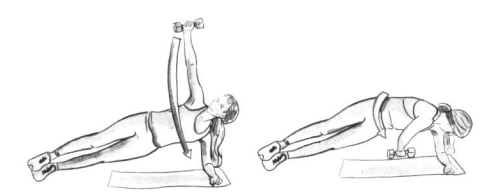

3b. Ski Mogul

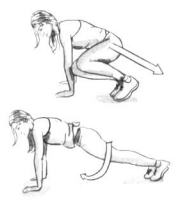

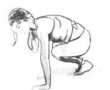

(Left Side) SET 1 REPS: _____ → SET 1 REPS: _____

(Right Side) SET 2 REPS: _____ → SET 2 REPS: _____

(Alternate Sides) SET 3 REPS: _____ → SET 3 REPS: _____

---

30 SECOND BREAK

CIRCUIT 4
(30s EACH)

4a. Burpee

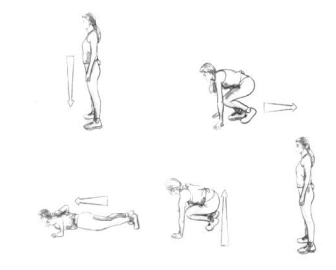

SET 1 REPS: _____ → (15s) REST

SET 2 REPS: _____ → (15s) REST

SET 3 REPS: _____ → (15s) REST

SET 4 REPS: _____ → (15s) REST

---

30 SECOND BREAK

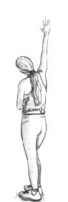

COOL DOWN
(60s EACH)

a. Lat Stretch   **b. Glute Stretch**   **c. Pigeon Stretch**   **d. Runner's Stretch**

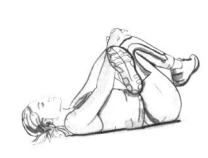

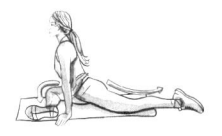

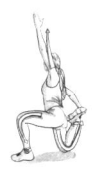

TODAY'S WORKOUT INTENSITY: _____ / 10

EXERCISE GUIDE
https://HabitNest.link/booty18

Workout 18: Resistance Training

DATE: _____

1. Squat

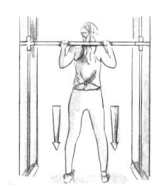

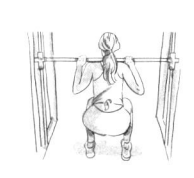

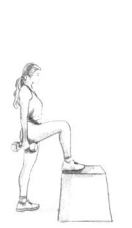

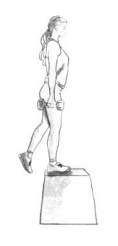

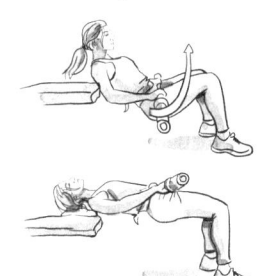

SET 1	REPS: _____ (GOAL: 15-20)	WEIGHT: _____
SET 2	REPS: _____ (GOAL: 12-15)	WEIGHT: _____
SET 3	REPS: _____ (GOAL: 10-12)	WEIGHT: _____
SET 4 (Optional)	REPS: _____ (GOAL: 8-10)	WEIGHT: _____

2. Alternating Step Up

SET 1	REPS: _____ (GOAL: 15-20)	WEIGHT: _____
SET 2	REPS: _____ (GOAL: 12-15)	WEIGHT: _____
SET 3	REPS: _____ (GOAL: 10-12)	WEIGHT: _____
SET 4 (Optional)	REPS: _____ (GOAL: 8-10)	WEIGHT: _____

3. Hip Thrust

SET 1	REPS: _____ (GOAL: 15-20)	WEIGHT: _____
SET 2	REPS: _____ (GOAL: 12-15)	WEIGHT: _____
SET 3	REPS: _____ (GOAL: 10-12)	WEIGHT: _____
SET 4 (Optional)	REPS: _____ (GOAL: 8-10)	WEIGHT: _____

4. Single Leg Deadlift

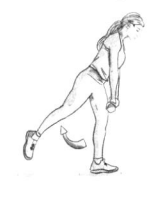

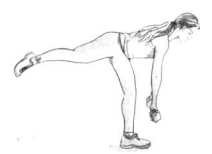

Left | Right

SET 1	REPS: ___	___ (GOAL: 15-20)	WEIGHT: _____
SET 2	REPS: ___	___ (GOAL: 12-15)	WEIGHT: _____
SET 3	REPS: ___	___ (GOAL: 10-12)	WEIGHT: _____
SET 4 (Optional)	REPS: ___	___ (GOAL: 8-10)	WEIGHT: _____

TODAY'S WORKOUT INTENSITY: _____ / 10

EXERCISE GUIDE
https://HabitNest.link/booty19

Workout 19: 4-3-2-1

DATE _____

GLUTE ACTIVATION WARMUP
30s EACH

a. Clam Opener

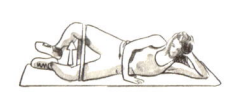

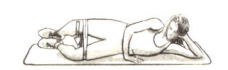

(30s Each Side)

b. Tabletop w/Donkey Kick

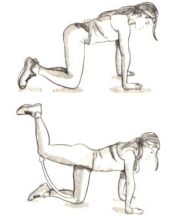

c. Glute Bridge w/ Band Flutter

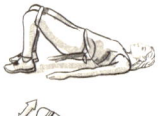

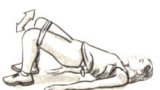

d. Lateral Leg Raise

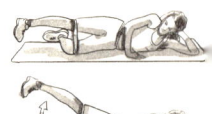

- 30s Each Leg (w/ Foot Flexed)
- 30s Each Leg (w/ Toes Pointing)

--- 30 SECOND BREAK ---

CIRCUIT 1
60s EACH

1a. Squat Thrust

REPS: _____ →

1b. Side to Side Squat

REPS: _____ →

1c. Fast Feet

REPS: _____ →

1d. Side Triangle Crunch

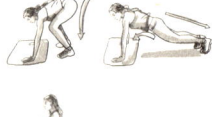

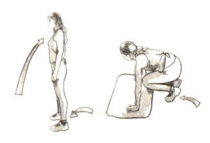

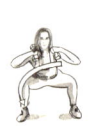

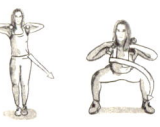

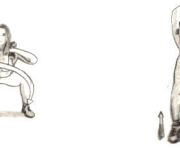

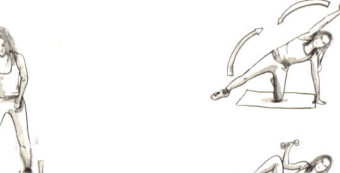

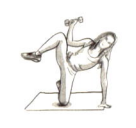

REPS: _____
(30s Each Side)

--- 30 SECOND BREAK ---

CIRCUIT 2
50s EACH

2a. Side V-Up

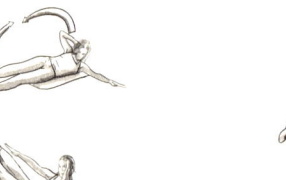

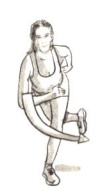

(Left Side) SET 1 REPS: _____ →
(Right Side) SET 2 REPS: _____ →

2b. Speed Skater

SET 1 REPS: _____ →
SET 2 REPS: _____ →

2c. Russian Twist

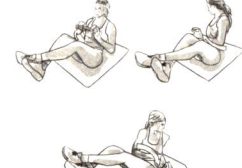

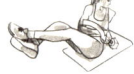

SET 1 REPS: _____
SET 2 REPS: _____

―――― 30 SECOND BREAK ――――

CIRCUIT 3
(40s EACH)

3a. 3-Point Lunge

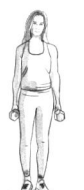

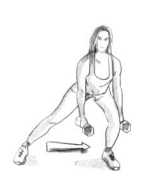

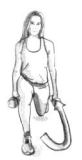

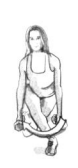

3b. Burpee

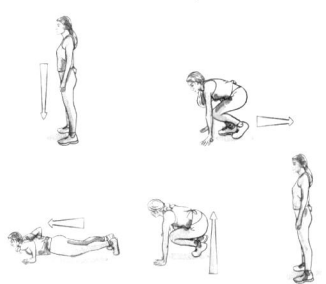

(Left Leg)   SET 1 REPS: _____ → SET 1 REPS: _____
(Right Leg)   SET 2 REPS: _____ → SET 2 REPS: _____
(Alternate Legs) SET 3 REPS: _____ → SET 3 REPS: _____

―――― 30 SECOND BREAK ――――

CIRCUIT 4
(30s EACH)

4a. The Heisman

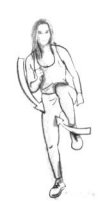

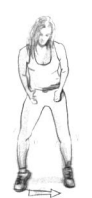

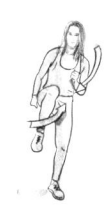

SET 1 REPS: _____ → 15s REST
SET 2 REPS: _____ → 15s REST
SET 3 REPS: _____ → 15s REST
SET 4 REPS: _____ → 15s REST

―――― 30 SECOND BREAK ――――

COOL DOWN
(60s EACH)

a. Pigeon Stretch   **b. Crossbody Hangover**   **c. Glute Stretch**   **d. Butterfly Stretch**

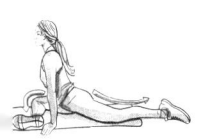

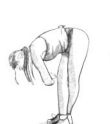

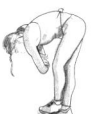

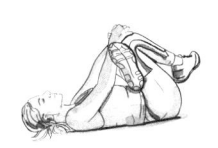

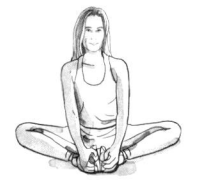

TODAY'S WORKOUT INTENSITY: _____ / 10

Workout 20: Resistance Training

DATE _____

https://HabitNest.link/booty20

1. Cable Row w/Squat

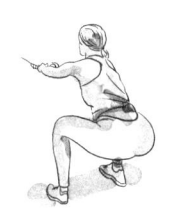

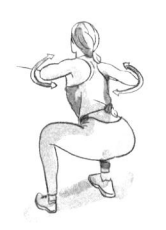

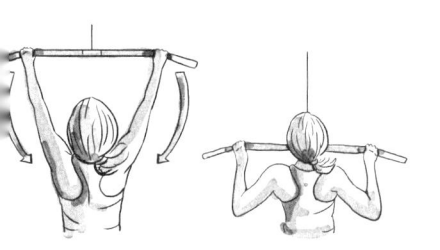

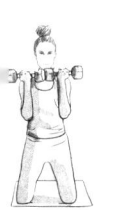

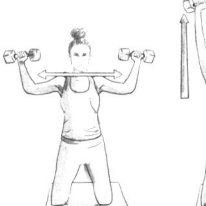

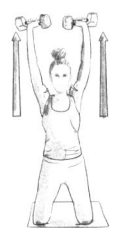

SET 1	REPS: _____ (GOAL: 15-20)	WEIGHT: _____
SET 2	REPS: _____ (GOAL: 12-15)	WEIGHT: _____
SET 3	REPS: _____ (GOAL: 10-12)	WEIGHT: _____
SET 4 (Optional)	REPS: _____ (GOAL: 8-10)	WEIGHT: _____

2. Lat Pulldown

SET 1	REPS: _____ (GOAL: 15-20)	WEIGHT: _____
SET 2	REPS: _____ (GOAL: 12-15)	WEIGHT: _____
SET 3	REPS: _____ (GOAL: 10-12)	WEIGHT: _____
SET 4 (Optional)	REPS: _____ (GOAL: 8-10)	WEIGHT: _____

3. Arnold Press

SET 1	REPS: _____ (GOAL: 15-20)	WEIGHT: _____
SET 2	REPS: _____ (GOAL: 12-15)	WEIGHT: _____
SET 3	REPS: _____ (GOAL: 10-12)	WEIGHT: _____
SET 4 (Optional)	REPS: _____ (GOAL: 8-10)	WEIGHT: _____

4. Squat

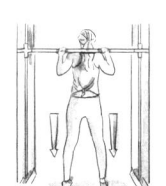

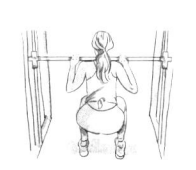

SET 1	REPS: _____ (GOAL: 15-20)	WEIGHT: _____
SET 2	REPS: _____ (GOAL: 12-15)	WEIGHT: _____
SET 3	REPS: _____ (GOAL: 10-12)	WEIGHT: _____
SET 4 (Optional)	REPS: _____ (GOAL: 8-10)	WEIGHT: _____

TODAY'S WORKOUT INTENSITY: _____ / 10

Check-In

How am I ACTUALLY feeling physically?

_____
_____
_____
_____

How am I feeling about the quality and intensity of my workouts? Can I do more or am I pushing the limit consistently? Am I getting enough rest?

_____
_____
_____
_____

How do I feel about the way I look? Do I see how much I can change if I stick to this program?

_____
_____
_____
_____

Am I mentally stronger?

_____
_____
_____
_____

Bonus Challenge

> *Achieve crazy mind-muscle connection with every single rep you perform.*

This bonus challenge specifically applies to resistance training days.

Many people understand mind-muscle connection as simply 'being focused' and 'not being distracted' during workouts. Although that's part of it, the true effectiveness of mind-muscle connection comes when you:

1. **Turn off all other muscles that are not part of the movement.** Only lift the weight using the specific muscles needed for it.

2. **Keep the muscle(s) you're using fully engaged, flexed, and isolated the entire time** throughout each movement. For every second of every rep.

To take this concept to the next level, you should isolate and flex the specific muscle you're going to use before every single exercise so you'll know exactly what to activate with each rep.

This means at the top or bottom of each rep, you keep your muscle engaged and fully lifting the weight as you would in the middle of a rep.

You may have to drastically drop in weight to do this, which is a sign you're doing a substantial amount of 'cheating reps' and leaving lots of a movement's primary muscles barely used.

You should also be prepared to know what muscles can help you break form and cheat so you can be extra vigilant of not using them.

Play around with this concept during your next workout if it's new for you and see if you notice a big difference.

Workout 21: 4-3-2-1

EXERCISE GUIDE
https://HabitNest.link/booty21

DATE _____

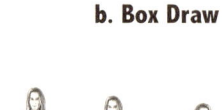

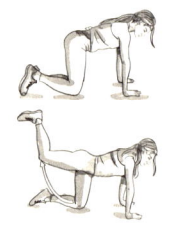

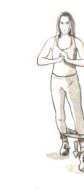

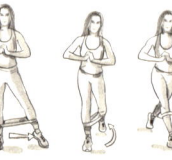

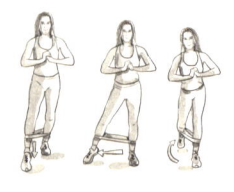

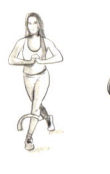

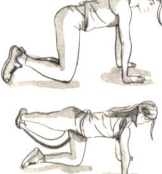

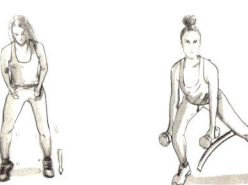

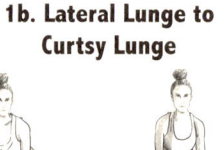

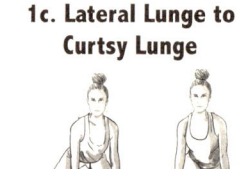

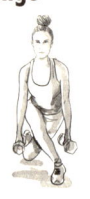

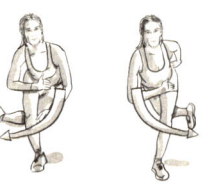

GLUTE ACTIVATION WARMUP
30s EACH

a. Tabletop w/ Donkey Kick
(30s Each Leg)

b. Box Draw
(Left Side)

c. Box Draw
(Right Side)

d. Tabletop w/ Diagonal Kick
(30s Each Leg)

— 30 SECOND BREAK —

CIRCUIT 1
60s EACH

1a. Fast Feet
REPS: _____

→ **1b. Lateral Lunge to Curtsy Lunge**
REPS: _____
(Left Side)

→ **1c. Lateral Lunge to Curtsy Lunge**
REPS: _____
(Right Side)

→ **1d. Speed Skater**
REPS: _____

— 30 SECOND BREAK —

CIRCUIT 2
50s EACH

2a. Plank Jack
SET 1 REPS: _____
SET 2 REPS: _____

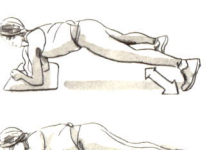

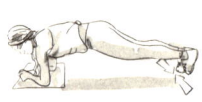

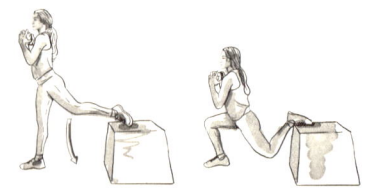

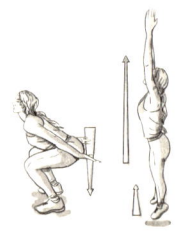

→ **2b. Bulgarian Lunge**
(Left Side) SET 1 REPS: _____
(Right Side) SET 2 REPS: _____

→ **2c. Vertical Leap**
SET 1 REPS: _____
SET 2 REPS: _____

── 30 SECOND BREAK ──

CIRCUIT 3
40s EACH

3a. Woodchopper ### 3b. Roundhouse Kick to Squat

(Left Leg)   SET 1 REPS: _____ → (Left Leg)   SET 1 REPS: _____
(Right Leg)   SET 2 REPS: _____ → (Right Leg)   SET 2 REPS: _____
(Alternate Legs) SET 3 REPS: _____ → (Alternate Legs) SET 3 REPS: _____

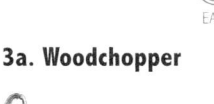

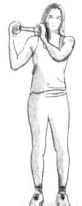

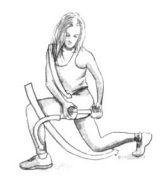

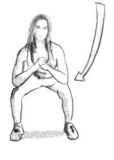

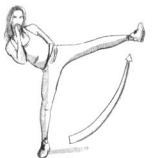

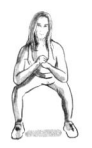

── 30 SECOND BREAK ──

CIRCUIT 4
30s EACH

4a. Leap Forward in Squat, Burpee, & Shuffle Back

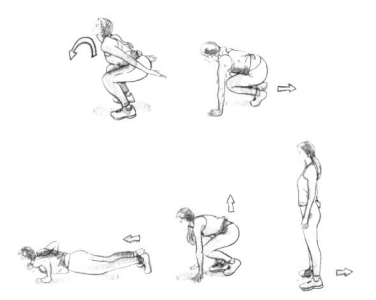

SET 1 REPS: _____ → 15s REST
SET 2 REPS: _____ → 15s REST
SET 3 REPS: _____ → 15s REST
SET 4 REPS: _____ → 15s REST

── 30 SECOND BREAK ──

COOL DOWN
60s EACH

a. Hamstring Stretch   **b. Runner's Stretch**   **c. Pigeon Stretch**   **d. Crossbody Hangover**

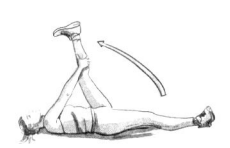

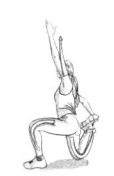

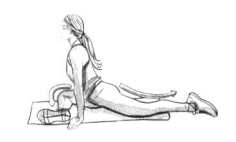

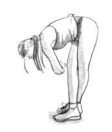

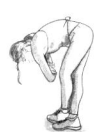

TODAY'S WORKOUT INTENSITY: _____ / 10

Workout 22: 4-3-2-1

EXERCISE GUIDE
https://HabitNest.link/booty22

DATE _____

GLUTE ACTIVATION WARMUP
30s EACH

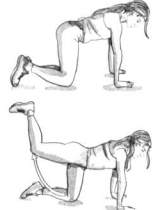

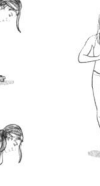

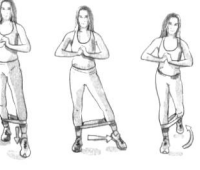

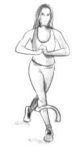

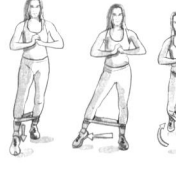

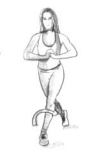

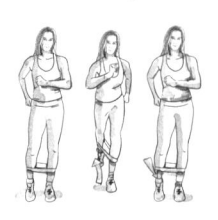

a. Tabletop w/ Donkey Kick
(30s Each Leg)

b. Box Draw
(Left Side)

c. Box Draw
(Right Side)

d. Running Man
(30s Each Side)

---— 30 SECOND BREAK ———

CIRCUIT 1
60s EACH

1a. Plank to Row

1b. Leg Drop

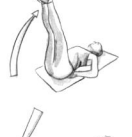

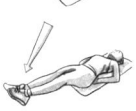

1c. Plie Squat w/ Shoulder Windmill

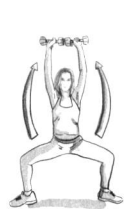

1d. Spider-Man Plank Crunch

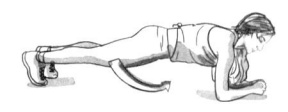

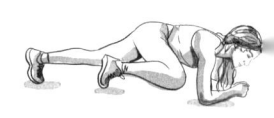

REPS: _____ (Alternate Arms) → REPS: _____ → REPS: _____ → REPS: _____ (Alternate Sides)

———— 30 SECOND BREAK ————

CIRCUIT 2
50s EACH

2a. 180° Jump Twist to Floor Tap

2b. Starfish Crunch

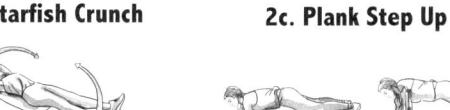

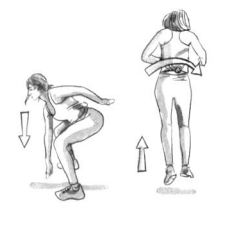

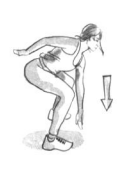

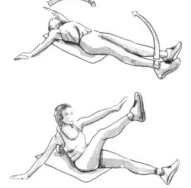

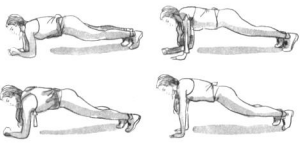

2c. Plank Step Up

SET 1 REPS: _____ → SET 1 REPS: _____ (Alternate Sides) → SET 1 REPS: _____ (Alternate Arms)

SET 2 REPS: _____ → SET 2 REPS: _____ (Alternate Sides) → SET 2 REPS: _____ (Alternate Arms)

100

― 30 SECOND BREAK ―

CIRCUIT 3
40s EACH

3a. 4 Donkey Kicks to 4 High Knees

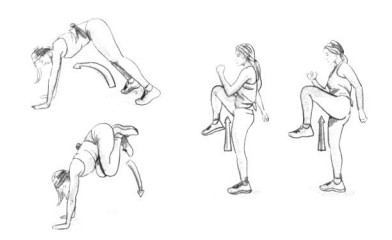

3b. Lateral Lunge w/ Knee to Elbow Rotation

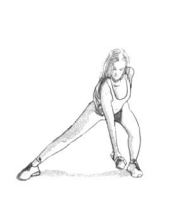

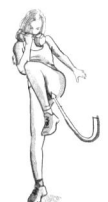

SET 1 REPS: _____ → (Left Leg) SET 1 REPS: _____

SET 2 REPS: _____ → (Right Leg) SET 2 REPS: _____

SET 3 REPS: _____ → (Alternate Legs) SET 3 REPS: _____

― 30 SECOND BREAK ―

CIRCUIT 4
30s EACH

4a. Burpee

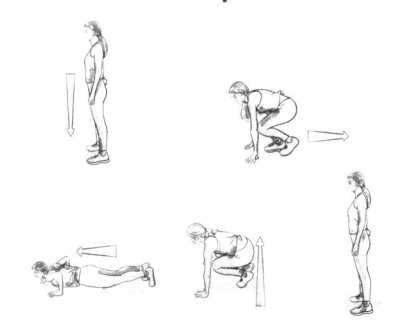

SET 1 REPS: _____ → 15s REST

SET 2 REPS: _____ → 15s REST

SET 3 REPS: _____ → 15s REST

SET 4 REPS: _____ → 15s REST

― 30 SECOND BREAK ―

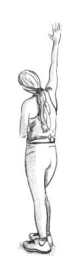

COOL DOWN
60s EACH

a. Lat Stretch   **b. Glute Stretch**   **c. Pigeon Stretch**   **d. Butterfly Stretch**

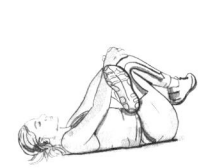

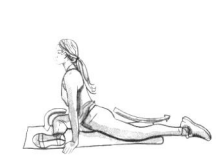

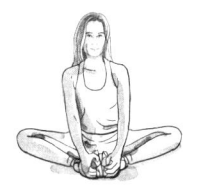

TODAY'S WORKOUT INTENSITY: _____ / 10

Workout 23: Resistance Training

DATE _____

1. Deadlift

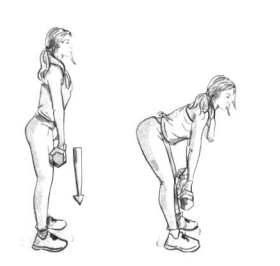

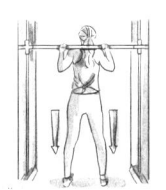

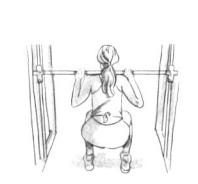

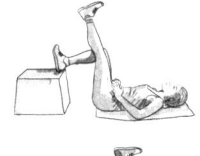

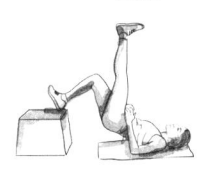

SET 1	REPS: _____	(GOAL: 15-20)	WEIGHT: _____
SET 2	REPS: _____	(GOAL: 12-15)	WEIGHT: _____
SET 3	REPS: _____	(GOAL: 10-12)	WEIGHT: _____
SET 4 (Optional)	REPS: _____	(GOAL: 8-10)	WEIGHT: _____

2. Squat

SET 1	REPS: _____	(GOAL: 15-20)	WEIGHT: _____
SET 2	REPS: _____	(GOAL: 12-15)	WEIGHT: _____
SET 3	REPS: _____	(GOAL: 10-12)	WEIGHT: _____
SET 4 (Optional)	REPS: _____	(GOAL: 8-10)	WEIGHT: _____

3. Single Leg Glute Bridge

SET 1	REPS: _____	(GOAL: 15-20)	WEIGHT: _____
SET 2	REPS: _____	(GOAL: 12-15)	WEIGHT: _____
SET 3	REPS: _____	(GOAL: 10-12)	WEIGHT: _____
SET 4 (Optional)	REPS: _____	(GOAL: 8-10)	WEIGHT: _____

4. Alternating Step Up

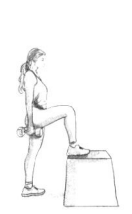

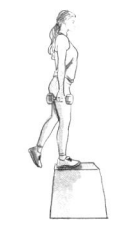

SET 1	REPS: _____	(GOAL: 15-20)	WEIGHT: _____
SET 2	REPS: _____	(GOAL: 12-15)	WEIGHT: _____
SET 3	REPS: _____	(GOAL: 10-12)	WEIGHT: _____
SET 4 (Optional)	REPS: _____	(GOAL: 8-10)	WEIGHT: _____

TODAY'S WORKOUT INTENSITY: _____ / 10

EXERCISE GUIDE
https://HabitNest.link/booty23

EXERCISE GUIDE
https://HabitNest.link/booty24

Workout 24: 4-3-2-1

DATE

GLUTE ACTIVATION WARMUP
(30s EACH)

a. Double Walk Out

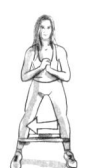

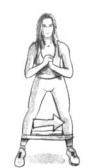

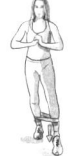

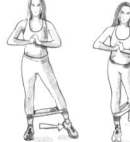

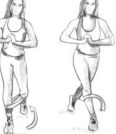

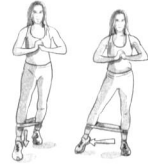

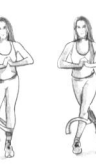

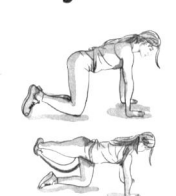

(2 Steps Right, 2 Steps Left)

b. Box Draw

(Left Leg)

c. Box Draw

(Right Leg)

d. Tabletop w/ Diagonal Kick

(30s Each Leg)

— 30 SECOND BREAK —

CIRCUIT 1
(60s EACH)

1a. Plank Jack

1b. V-Up

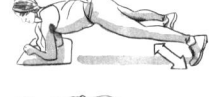

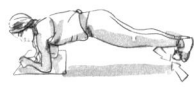

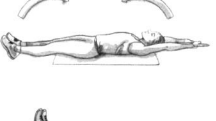

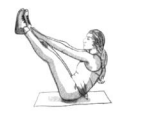

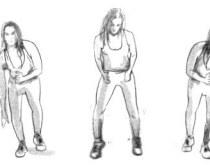

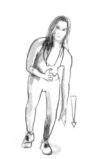

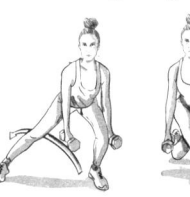

1c. Side Shuffle w/ Floor Tap

1d. Lateral Lunge to Curtsy Lunge

REPS: _____ → REPS: _____ → REPS: _____ → REPS: _____
(30s Each Side)

— 30 SECOND BREAK —

CIRCUIT 2
(50s EACH)

2a. Squat Thrust

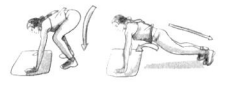

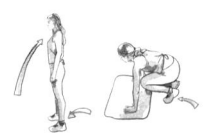

2b. Tabletop Elbow to Knee Crunch

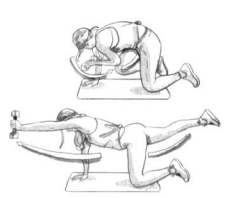

2c. Tabletop Elbow to Knee Crunch

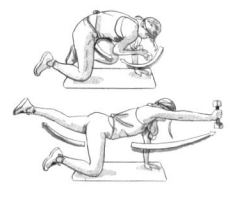

SET 1 REPS: _____ → SET 1 REPS: _____ → SET 1 REPS: _____
                        (Right Knee to Left Elbow)   (Left Knee to Right Elbow)

SET 2 REPS: _____ → SET 2 REPS: _____ → SET 2 REPS: _____
                        (Right Knee to Left Elbow)   (Left Knee to Right Elbow)

104

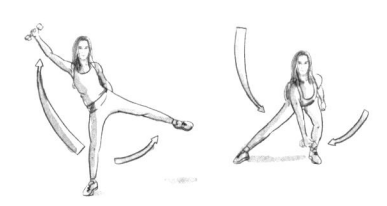

---– 30 SECOND BREAK ---–

CIRCUIT 3
40s EACH

3a. Lateral Lunge w/ Half 'X'   ### 3b. Mountain Climber

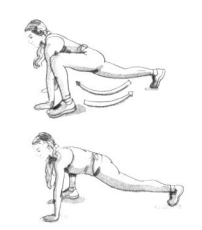

(Left Leg)   SET 1 REPS: _____ → SET 1 REPS: _____

(Right Leg)   SET 2 REPS: _____ → SET 2 REPS: _____

(Alternate Legs) SET 3 REPS: _____ → SET 3 REPS: _____

---– 30 SECOND BREAK ---–

CIRCUIT 4
30s EACH

4a. Burpee

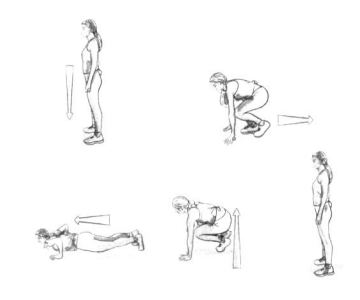

SET 1 REPS: _____ → 15s REST

SET 2 REPS: _____ → 15s REST

SET 3 REPS: _____ → 15s REST

SET 4 REPS: _____ → 15s REST

---– 30 SECOND BREAK ---–

COOL DOWN
60s EACH

a. Hamstring Stretch   **b. Butterfly Stretch**   **c. Glute Stretch**   **d. Crossbody Hangover**

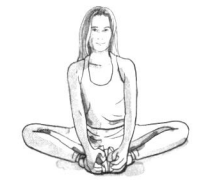

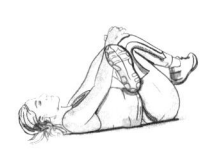

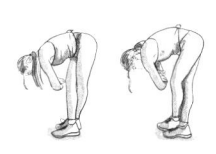

TODAY'S WORKOUT INTENSITY: _____ / 10

Workout 25: Resistance Training

DATE _____

https://HabitNest.link/booty25

1. Reverse Dumbbell Fly

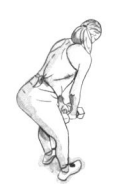

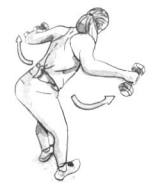

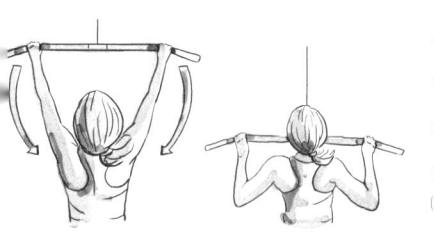

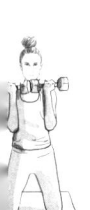

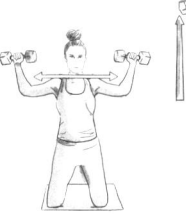

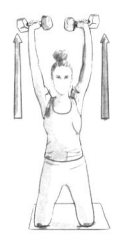

SET 1	REPS: _____	(GOAL: 15-20)	WEIGHT: _____
SET 2	REPS: _____	(GOAL: 12-15)	WEIGHT: _____
SET 3	REPS: _____	(GOAL: 10-12)	WEIGHT: _____
SET 4 (Optional)	REPS: _____	(GOAL: 8-10)	WEIGHT: _____

2. Lat Pulldown

SET 1	REPS: _____	(GOAL: 15-20)	WEIGHT: _____
SET 2	REPS: _____	(GOAL: 12-15)	WEIGHT: _____
SET 3	REPS: _____	(GOAL: 10 12)	WEIGHT: _____
SET 4 (Optional)	REPS: _____	(GOAL: 8-10)	WEIGHT: _____

3. Arnold Press

SET 1	REPS: _____	(GOAL: 15-20)	WEIGHT: _____
SET 2	REPS: _____	(GOAL: 12-15)	WEIGHT: _____
SET 3	REPS: _____	(GOAL: 10-12)	WEIGHT: _____
SET 4 (Optional)	REPS: _____	(GOAL: 8-10)	WEIGHT: _____

4. Cable Row w/Squat

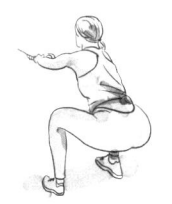

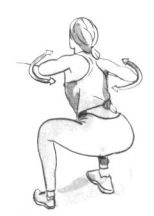

SET 1	REPS: _____	(GOAL: 15-20)	WEIGHT: _____
SET 2	REPS: _____	(GOAL: 12-15)	WEIGHT: _____
SET 3	REPS: _____	(GOAL: 10-12)	WEIGHT: _____
SET 4 (Optional)	REPS: _____	(GOAL: 8-10)	WEIGHT: _____

TODAY'S WORKOUT INTENSITY: _____ / 10

EXERCISE GUIDE
https://HabitNest.link/booty26

Workout 26: 4-3-2-1

DATE: _____

GLUTE ACTIVATION WARMUP
30s EACH

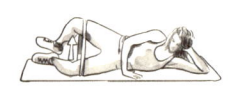

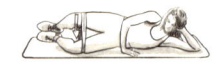

a. Clam Opener
(30s Each Leg)

b. Glute Bridge w/ Leg Extension
(30s Each Leg)

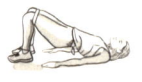

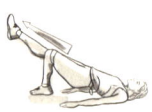

c. Double Walk Out
(2 Steps Right, 2 Steps Left)

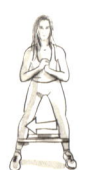

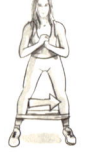

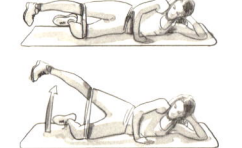

d. Lateral Leg Raise
- 30s Each Leg (w/ Foot Flexed)
- 30s Each Leg (w/ Toes Pointing Down)

--- 30 SECOND BREAK ---

CIRCUIT 1
60s EACH

1a. Mountain Climber
REPS: _____
(Alternate Legs)

→ **1b. 3-Point Lunge**
REPS: _____
(Left Leg)

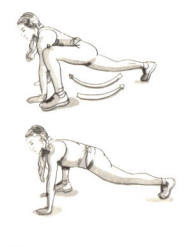

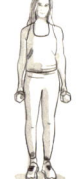

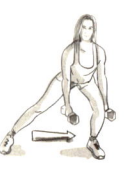

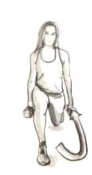

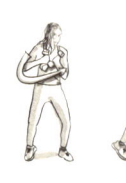

→ **1c. 3-Point Lunge**
REPS: _____
(Right Leg)

→ **1d. Boxing Jab**
REPS: _____

--- 30 SECOND BREAK ---

CIRCUIT 2
50s EACH

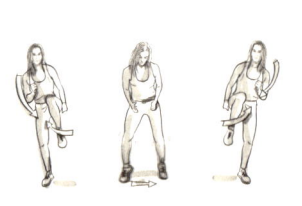

2a. The Heisman
SET 1 REPS: _____
SET 2 REPS: _____

→ **2b. Pendulum Lunge**
SET 1 REPS: _____
SET 2 REPS: _____

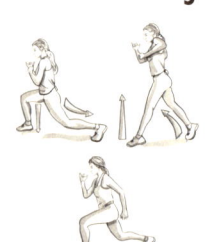

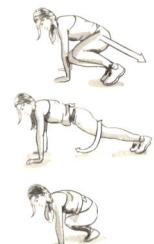

→ **2c. Ski Mogul**
SET 1 REPS: _____
SET 2 REPS: _____

―――――― 30 SECOND BREAK ――――――

CIRCUIT 3
40s EACH

3a. Lateral Lunge to Curtsy Lunge

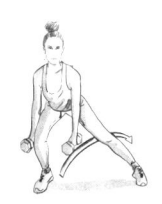

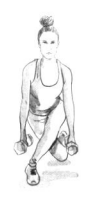

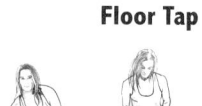

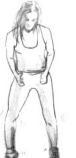

3b. Side Shuffle w/ Floor Tap

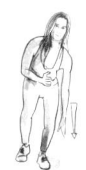

(Left Leg)   SET 1 REPS: _____ → SET 1 REPS: _____

(Right Leg)   SET 2 REPS: _____ → SET 2 REPS: _____

(Alternate Legs) SET 3 REPS: _____ → SET 3 REPS: _____

―――――― 30 SECOND BREAK ――――――

CIRCUIT 4
30s EACH

4a. Jump Squat

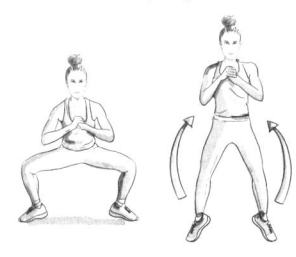

SET 1 REPS: _____ → 15s REST

SET 2 REPS: _____ → 15s REST

SET 3 REPS: _____ → 15s REST

SET 4 REPS: _____ → 15s REST

―――――― 30 SECOND BREAK ――――――

COOL DOWN
60s EACH

a. Hamstring Stretch **b. Pigeon Stretch** **c. Lat Stretch** **d. Runner's Stretch**

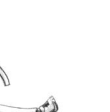

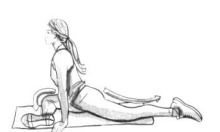

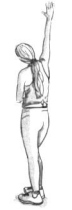

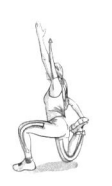

TODAY'S WORKOUT INTENSITY: _____ / 10

EXERCISE GUIDE
https://HabitNest.link/booty27

Workout 27: 4-3-2-1

DATE _____

GLUTE ACTIVATION WARMUP
(30s EACH)

a. Clam Opener
(30s Each Side)

b. Glute Bridge w/ Leg Extension
(Right Leg)

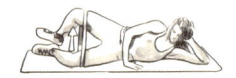

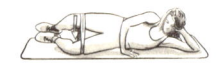

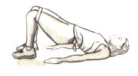

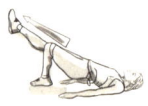

c. Glute Bridge w/ Leg Extension
(Left Leg)

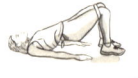

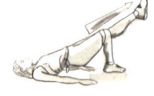

d. Lateral Leg Raise
- 30s Each Leg (w/ Foot Flexed)
- 30s Each Leg (w/ Toes Pointing Down)

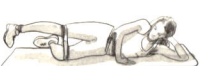

--- 30 SECOND BREAK ---

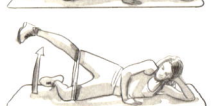

CIRCUIT 1
(60s EACH)

1a. Squat Thrust
REPS: _____ →

1b. Standing Side Crunch
REPS: _____
(Right Side) →

1c. Standing Side Crunch
REPS: _____
(Left Side) →

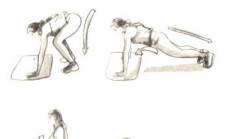

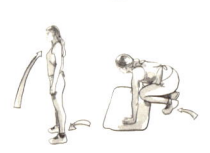

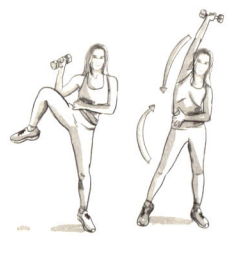

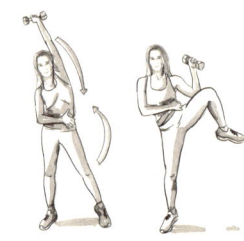

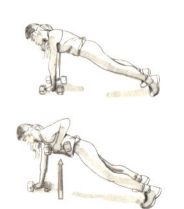

1d. Plank to Row
REPS: _____

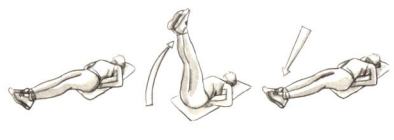

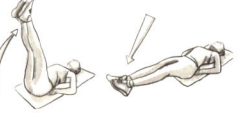

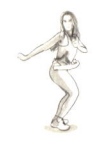

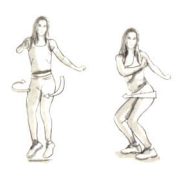

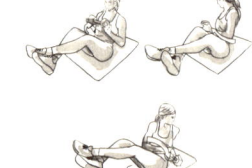

--- 30 SECOND BREAK ---

CIRCUIT 2
(50s EACH)

2a. Leg Drop
SET 1 REPS: _____ →
SET 2 REPS: _____ →

2b. Jump Twist
SET 1 REPS: _____
SET 2 REPS: _____ →

2c. Russian Twist
SET 1 REPS: _____
SET 2 REPS: _____

110

— 30 SECOND BREAK —

CIRCUIT 3
40s EACH

3a. Squat to Overhead Press

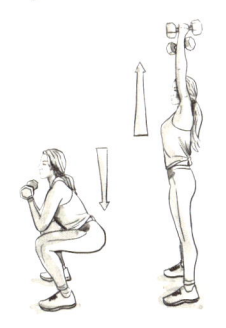

3b. Starfish Crunch

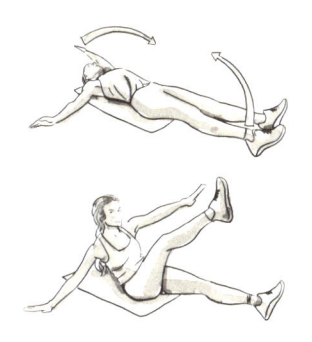

SET 1 REPS: _____ → (Alternate Sides) SET 1 REPS: _____

SET 2 REPS: _____ → (Alternate Sides) SET 2 REPS: _____

SET 3 REPS: _____ → (Alternate Sides) SET 3 REPS: _____

— 30 SECOND BREAK —

CIRCUIT 4
30s EACH

4a. 4 Donkey Kicks to 4 High Knees

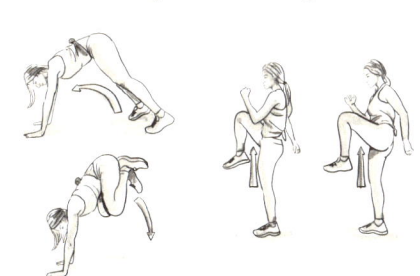

SET 1 REPS: _____ → 15s REST

SET 2 REPS: _____ → 15s REST

SET 3 REPS: _____ → 15s REST

SET 4 REPS: _____ → 15s REST

— 30 SECOND BREAK —

COOL DOWN
60s EACH

a. Glute Stretch   **b. Pigeon Stretch**   **c. Hamstring Stretch**   **d. Butterfly Stretch**

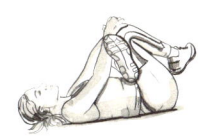

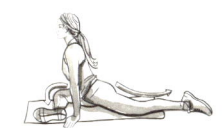

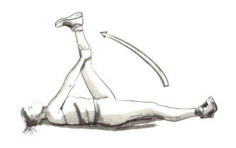

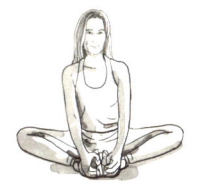

TODAY'S WORKOUT INTENSITY: _____ / 10

Workout 28: Resistance Training

DATE _____

1. Hip Thrust

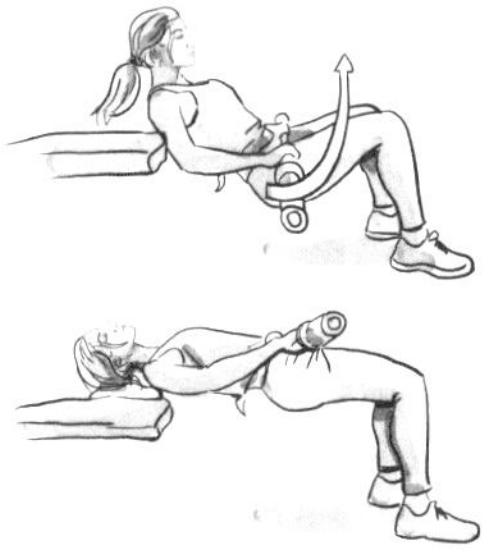

SET 1	REPS: _____	(GOAL: 15-20)	WEIGHT: _____
SET 2	REPS: _____	(GOAL: 12-15)	WEIGHT: _____
SET 3	REPS: _____	(GOAL: 10-12)	WEIGHT: _____
SET 4 (Optional)	REPS: _____	(GOAL: 8-10)	WEIGHT: _____

2. Squat

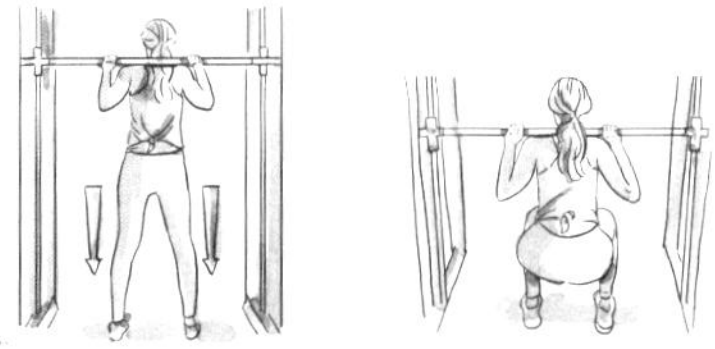

SET 1	REPS: _____	(GOAL: 15-20)	WEIGHT: _____
SET 2	REPS: _____	(GOAL: 12-15)	WEIGHT: _____
SET 3	REPS: _____	(GOAL: 10-12)	WEIGHT: _____
SET 4 (Optional)	REPS: _____	(GOAL: 8-10)	WEIGHT: _____

3. Elevated Plie Squat

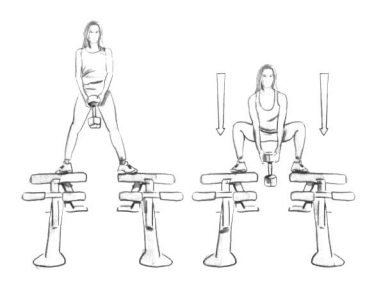

SET 1	REPS: _____	(GOAL: 15-20)	WEIGHT: _____
SET 2	REPS: _____	(GOAL: 12-15)	WEIGHT: _____
SET 3	REPS: _____	(GOAL: 10-12)	WEIGHT: _____
SET 4 (Optional)	REPS: _____	(GOAL: 8-10)	WEIGHT: _____

4. Deadlift

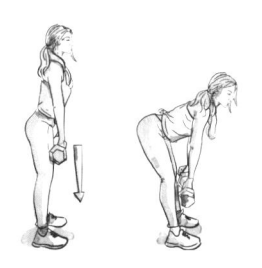

SET 1	REPS: _____	(GOAL: 15-20)	WEIGHT: _____
SET 2	REPS: _____	(GOAL: 12-15)	WEIGHT: _____
SET 3	REPS: _____	(GOAL: 10-12)	WEIGHT: _____
SET 4 (Optional)	REPS: _____	(GOAL: 8-10)	WEIGHT: _____

EXERCISE GUIDE
https://HabitNest.link/booty28

TODAY'S WORKOUT INTENSITY: _____ / 10

EXERCISE GUIDE
https://HabitNest.link/booty29

Workout 29: 4-3-2-1

DATE _____

GLUTE ACTIVATION WARMUP
(30s EACH)

a. Clam Opener

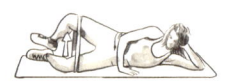

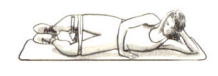

b. Tabletop w/ Donkey Kick

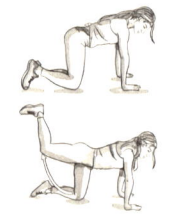

c. Glute Bridge w/ Leg Extension

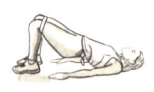

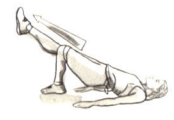

d. Fire Hydrant

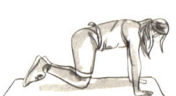

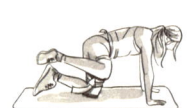

(30s Each Side) (30s Each Side) (30s Each Side) (30s Each Side)

— 30 SECOND BREAK —

CIRCUIT 1
(60s EACH)

1a. Leap Forward In Squat, Burpee, & Shuffle Back

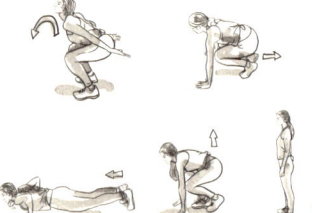

1b. Side Triangle Crunch

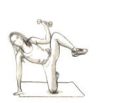

1c. Side Triangle Crunch

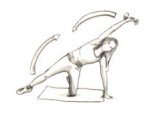

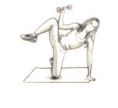

1d. Fast Feet

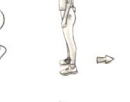

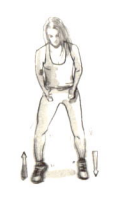

REPS: _____ → REPS: _____ → REPS: _____ → REPS: _____
                   (Left Side)   (Right Side)

— 30 SECOND BREAK —

CIRCUIT 2
(50s EACH)

2a. Roundhouse Kick to Squat

2b. Side Plank w/ Elbow Twist

2c. Ski Mogul

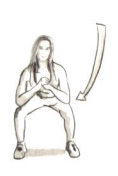

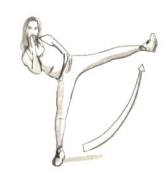

SET 1 REPS: _____ → SET 1 REPS: _____ → SET 1 REPS: _____
(Right Leg)   (Right Side)

SET 2 REPS: _____ → SET 2 REPS: _____ → SET 2 REPS: _____
(Left Leg)   (Left Side)

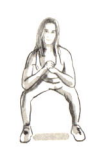

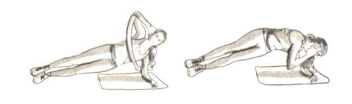

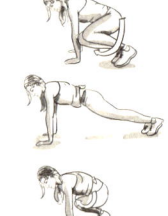

―――― 30 SECOND BREAK ――――

CIRCUIT 3
40s EACH

3a. Lateral Lunge to Curtsy Lunge

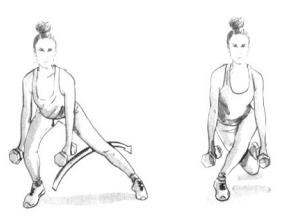

3b. Starfish Crunch

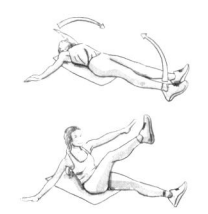

(Left Leg)	SET 1 REPS: _____	→	(Left Leg)	SET 1 REPS: _____
(Right Leg)	SET 2 REPS: _____	→	(Right Leg)	SET 2 REPS: _____
(Alternate Legs)	SET 3 REPS: _____	→	(Alternate Legs)	SET 3 REPS: _____

―――― 30 SECOND BREAK ――――

CIRCUIT 4
30s EACH

4a. Burpee

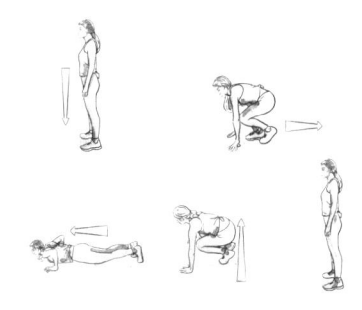

SET 1 REPS: _____ → 15s REST
SET 2 REPS: _____ → 15s REST
SET 3 REPS: _____ → 15s REST
SET 4 REPS: _____ → 15s REST

―――― 30 SECOND BREAK ――――

COOL DOWN
60s EACH

a. Pigeon Stretch   **b. Glute Stretch**   **c. Hamstring Stretch**   **d. Crossbody Hangover**

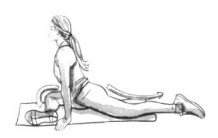

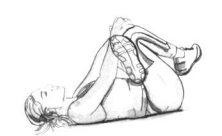

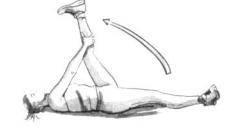

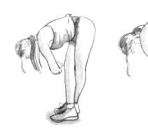

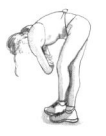

115   **TODAY'S WORKOUT INTENSITY:** _____ / 10

EXERCISE GUIDE
https://HabitNest.link/booty30

Workout 30: Resistance Training

DATE _____

1. Deadlift

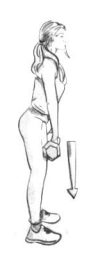

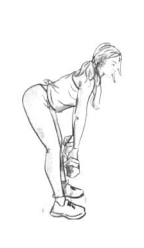

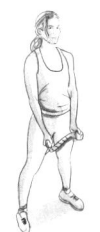

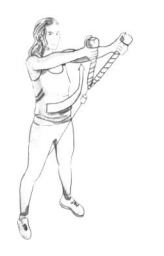

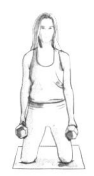

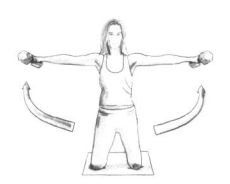

SET 1 REPS: _____ (GOAL: 15-20)	WEIGHT: _____
SET 2 REPS: _____ (GOAL: 12-15)	WEIGHT: _____
SET 3 REPS: _____ (GOAL: 10-12)	WEIGHT: _____
SET 4 REPS: _____ (GOAL: 8-10)	WEIGHT: _____
(Optional)

2. Shoulder Rope Pull

SET 1 REPS: _____ (GOAL: 15-20)   WEIGHT: _____
SET 2 REPS: _____ (GOAL: 12-15)   WEIGHT: _____
SET 3 REPS: _____ (GOAL: 10-12)   WEIGHT: _____
SET 4 REPS: _____ (GOAL: 8-10)   WEIGHT: _____
(Optional)

3. Lateral Raise

SET 1 REPS: _____ (GOAL: 15-20)   WEIGHT: _____
SET 2 REPS: _____ (GOAL: 12-15)   WEIGHT: _____
SET 3 REPS: _____ (GOAL: 10-12)   WEIGHT: _____
SET 4 REPS: _____ (GOAL: 8-10)   WEIGHT: _____
(Optional)

4. Hip Thrust

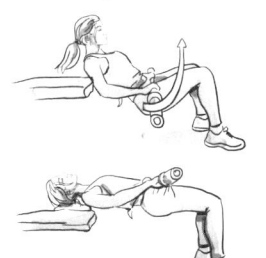

SET 1 REPS: _____ (GOAL: 15-20)   WEIGHT: _____
SET 2 REPS: _____ (GOAL: 12-15)   WEIGHT: _____
SET 3 REPS: _____ (GOAL: 10-12)   WEIGHT: _____
SET 4 REPS: _____ (GOAL: 8-10)   WEIGHT: _____
(Optional)

TODAY'S WORKOUT INTENSITY: _____ / 10

Check-In

How am I ACTUALLY feeling physically?

How am I feeling about the quality and intensity of my workouts? Can I do more or am I pushing the limit consistently? Am I getting enough rest?

How do I feel about the way I look?

Have people started mentioning anything about my physique? How can these comments be helpful? How might they be unhelpful?

Pro-Tip

> *Push for progressive overload week after week.*

You can achieve a new level of progressive overload in 3 different ways:

1. *Increase the weight you use*
2. *Increase the reps you do, or*
3. *Increase the speed/intensity you complete the workout in.*

You have to hit progressive overload in at least one of these ways in order to improve stamina, endurance, and keep challenging yourself.

On resistance training days, one effective way to build this as a habit is by doing one extra rep at the end of each set once you feel you've 'really hit failure.'

If you fail and can't do that extra rep, try holding / supporting the weight for as long as possible, even if it's a half-rep (and make sure it's safe to do so without injuring yourself). This will give you a crazy additional pump.

If you DO end up completing that additional rep, that's a huge win too as you're breaking into new levels of intensity. You'll also be learning that you may have extra fuel in the tank to push your workouts even harder. If you end up completing this extra rep, keep going to see if you can complete even more afterwards.

On 4-3-2-1 days, you should place a focus on increasing the number of reps you do for each exercise within the given time range or increase the speed and power you perform each rep.

Repeat this process as you progress through the journal.

Workout 31: 4-3-2-1

EXERCISE GUIDE
https://HabitNest.link/booty31

DATE _____

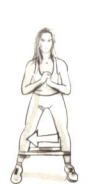

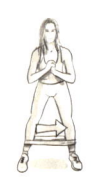

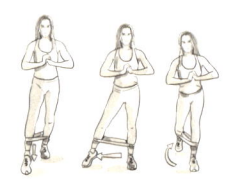

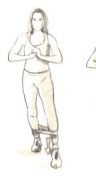

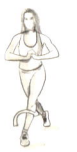

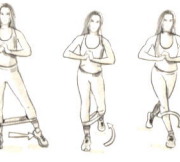

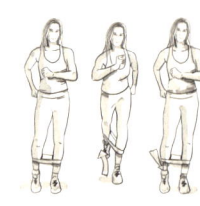

GLUTE ACTIVATION WARMUP
30s EACH

a. Double Walk Out **b. Box Draw** **c. Box Draw** **d. Running Man**

(2 Steps Right, 2 Steps Left)   (Right Leg)   (Left Leg)   (30s Each Leg)

--- 30 SECOND BREAK ---

CIRCUIT 1
60s EACH

1a. Burpee   **1b. Plie Squat w/ Shoulder Windmill**   **1c. Ski Mogul**   **1d. V-Up**

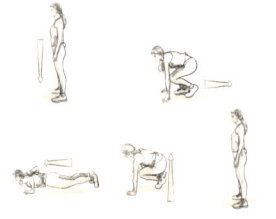

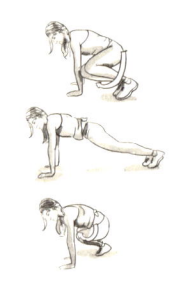

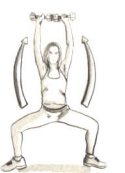

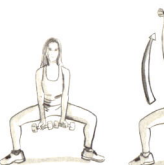

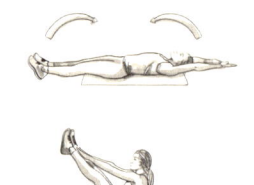

REPS: _____ → REPS: _____ → REPS: _____ → REPS: _____

--- 30 SECOND BREAK ---

CIRCUIT 2
50s EACH

2a. 4 Donkey Kicks to 4 High Knees   **2b. Pendulum Jack**   **2c. Lateral Lunge to Curtsy Lunge**

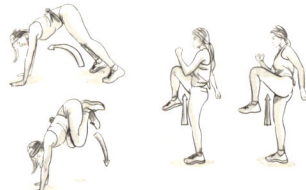

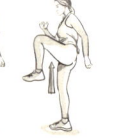

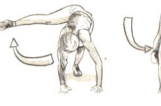

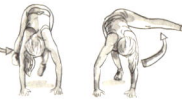

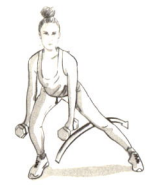

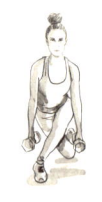

SET 1 REPS: _____ → SET 1 REPS: _____ → (Right Side) SET 1 REPS: _____

SET 2 REPS: _____ → SET 2 REPS: _____ → (Left Side) SET 2 REPS: _____

30 SECOND BREAK

CIRCUIT 3
40s EACH

3a. Plie Squat w/ Shoulder Windmill

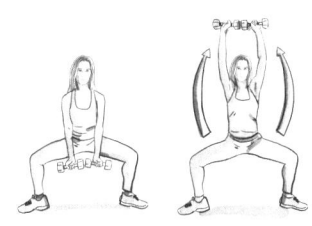

3b. Jump Squat

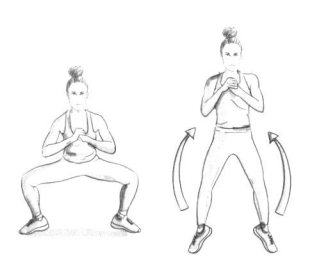

SET 1 REPS: _____ → SET 1 REPS: _____

SET 2 REPS: _____ → SET 2 REPS: _____

SET 3 REPS: _____ → SET 3 REPS: _____

30 SECOND BREAK

CIRCUIT 4
30s EACH

4a. In and Out Jack

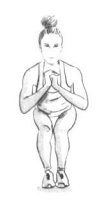

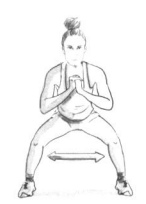

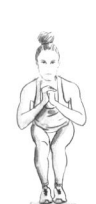

SET 1 REPS: _____ → 15s REST

SET 2 REPS: _____ → 15s REST

SET 3 REPS: _____ → 15s REST

SET 4 REPS: _____ → 15s REST

30 SECOND BREAK

COOL DOWN
60s EACH

a. Runner's Stretch   **b. Butterfly Stretch**   **c. Lat Stretch**   **d. Pigeon Stretch**

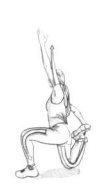

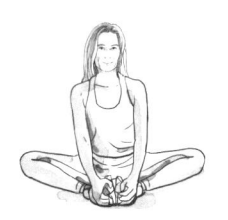

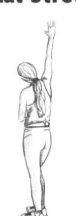

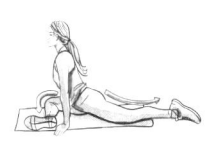

TODAY'S WORKOUT INTENSITY: _____ / 10

EXERCISE GUIDE
https://HabitNest.link/booty32

Workout 32: 4-3-2-1

DATE

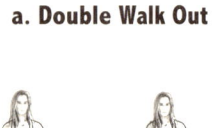

GLUTE ACTIVATION WARMUP
30s EACH

a. Double Walk Out
(2 Steps Right, 2 Steps Left)

b. Box Draw
(Left Leg)

c. Box Draw
(Right Leg)

d. Running Man
(30s Each Leg)

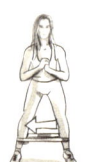

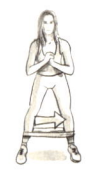

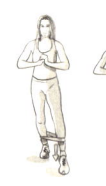

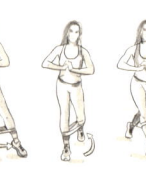

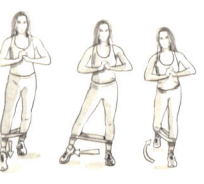

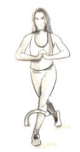

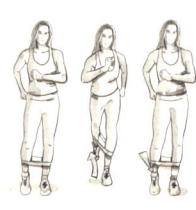

--- 30 SECOND BREAK ---

CIRCUIT 1
60s EACH

1a. Boxing Jab

1b. Plank Knee Tuck

1c. Vertical Sit-Up w/ Elbow to Knee Touch

1d. 180° Jump Twist to Floor Tap

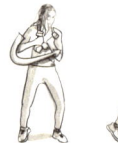

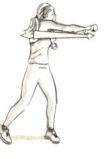

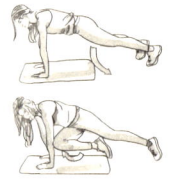

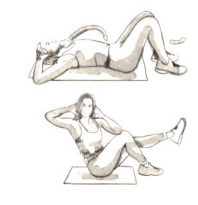

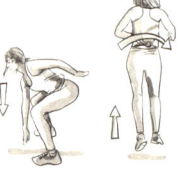

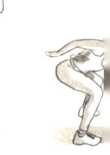

REPS: _____ → REPS: _____ (Alternate Sides) → REPS: _____ (Alternate Sides) → REPS: _____

--- 30 SECOND BREAK ---

CIRCUIT 2
50s EACH

2a. Leg Drop

2b. Squat Thrust

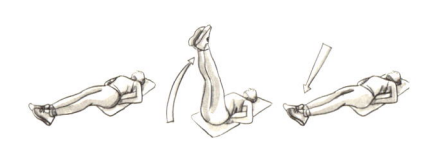

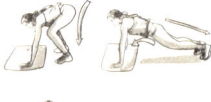

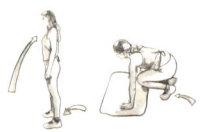

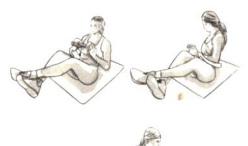

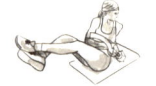

2c. Russian Twist

SET 1 REPS: _____ → SET 1 REPS: _____ → SET 1 REPS: _____

SET 2 REPS: _____ → SET 2 REPS: _____ → SET 2 REPS: _____

─── 30 SECOND BREAK ───

CIRCUIT 3
40s EACH

3a. Side Triangle Crunch　　　　### 3b. Jump Squat

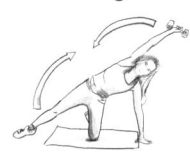

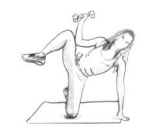

(Left Side)	SET 1 REPS: _____	→	SET 1 REPS: _____
(Right Side)	SET 2 REPS: _____	→	SET 2 REPS: _____
(Alternate Side)	SET 3 REPS: _____	→	SET 3 REPS: _____

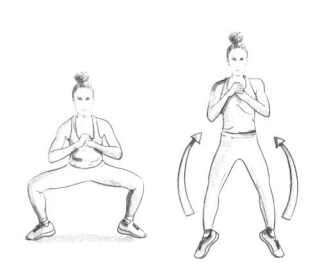

─── 30 SECOND BREAK ───

CIRCUIT 4
30s EACH

4a. Burpee

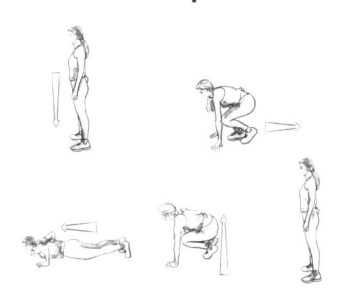

SET 1 REPS: _____ → 15s REST
SET 2 REPS: _____ → 15s REST
SET 3 REPS: _____ → 15s REST
SET 4 REPS: _____ → 15s REST

─── 30 SECOND BREAK ───

COOL DOWN
60s EACH

a. Butterfly Stretch　　**b. Hamstring Stretch**　　**c. Lat Stretch**　　**d. Glute Stretch**

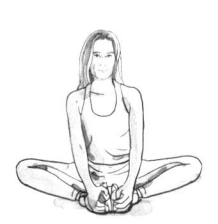

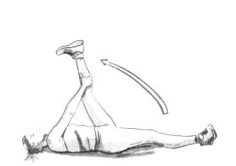

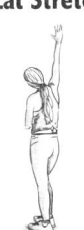

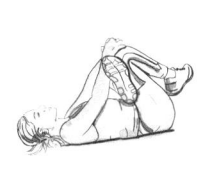

TODAY'S WORKOUT INTENSITY: _____ / 10

Workout 33: Resistance Training

DATE _____

https://HabitNest.link/booty33

1. Deadlift

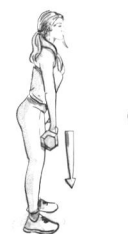

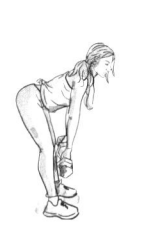

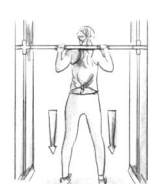

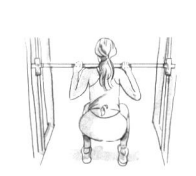

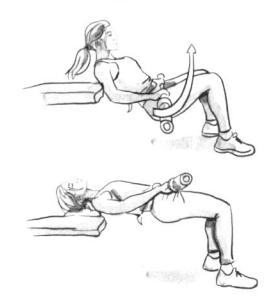

SET 1	REPS: _____	(GOAL: 15-20)	WEIGHT: _____
SET 2	REPS: _____	(GOAL: 12-15)	WEIGHT: _____
SET 3	REPS: _____	(GOAL: 10-12)	WEIGHT: _____
SET 4 (Optional)	REPS: _____	(GOAL: 8-10)	WEIGHT: _____

2. Squat

SET 1	REPS: _____	(GOAL: 15-20)	WEIGHT: _____
SET 2	REPS: _____	(GOAL: 12-15)	WEIGHT: _____
SET 3	REPS: _____	(GOAL: 10-12)	WEIGHT: _____
SET 4 (Optional)	REPS: _____	(GOAL: 8-10)	WEIGHT: _____

3. Hip Thrust

SET 1	REPS: _____	(GOAL: 15-20)	WEIGHT: _____
SET 2	REPS: _____	(GOAL: 12-15)	WEIGHT: _____
SET 3	REPS: _____	(GOAL: 10-12)	WEIGHT: _____
SET 4 (Optional)	REPS: _____	(GOAL: 8-10)	WEIGHT: _____

4. Woodchopper

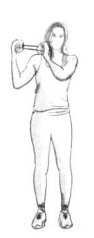

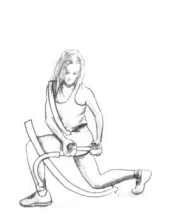

<u>Left</u> | <u>Right</u>

SET 1	REPS: _____	(GOAL: 15-20)	WEIGHT: _____
SET 2	REPS: _____	(GOAL: 12-15)	WEIGHT: _____
SET 3	REPS: _____	(GOAL: 10-12)	WEIGHT: _____
SET 4 (Optional)	REPS: _____	(GOAL: 8-10)	WEIGHT: _____

TODAY'S WORKOUT INTENSITY: _____ / 10

EXERCISE GUIDE
https://HabitNest.link/booty34

Workout 34: 4-3-2-1

DATE

GLUTE ACTIVATION WARMUP (30s EACH)

a. Tabletop w/ Diagonal Kick
(30s Each Leg)

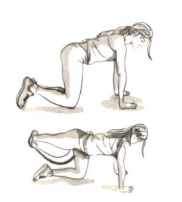

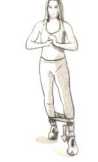

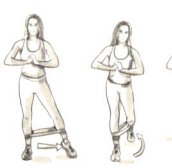

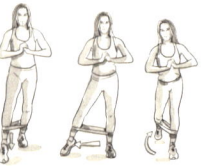

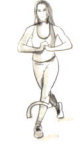

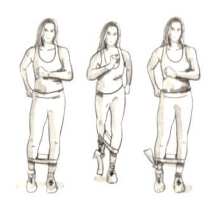

b. Box Draw
(Left Leg)

c. Box Draw
(Right Leg)

d. Running Man
(30s Each Leg)

--- 30 SECOND BREAK ---

CIRCUIT 1 (60s EACH)

1a. Squat Thrust → **1b. V-Up** → **1c. Side Shuffle w/ Floor Tap** → **1d. Russian Twist**

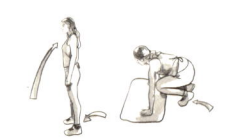

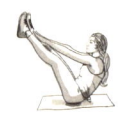

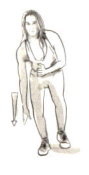

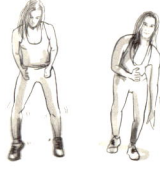

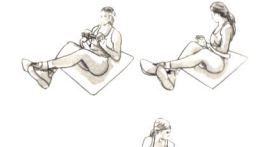

REPS: _____ → REPS: _____ → REPS: _____ → REPS: _____

--- 30 SECOND BREAK ---

CIRCUIT 2 (50s EACH)

2a. Lateral Lunge w/ Half-X → **2b. Tabletop Elbow to Knee Crunch** → **2c. Speed Skater**

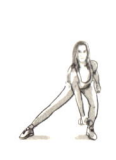

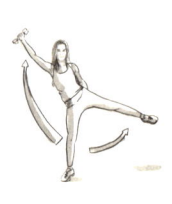

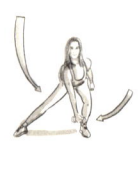

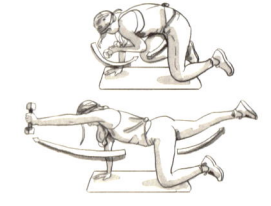

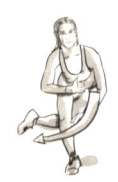

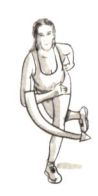

(Right Side) SET 1 REPS: _____ → SET 1 REPS: _____ → SET 1 REPS: _____
  (Right to Left)
(Left Side) SET 2 REPS: _____ → SET 2 REPS: _____ → SET 2 REPS: _____
  (Left to Right)

---- 30 SECOND BREAK ----

CIRCUIT 3
40s EACH

3a. Lateral Lunge to Curtsy Lunge

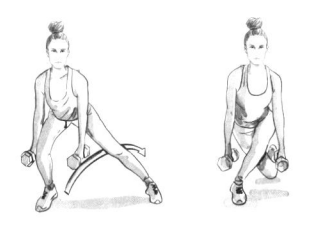

3b. Side Plank w/ Torso Twist

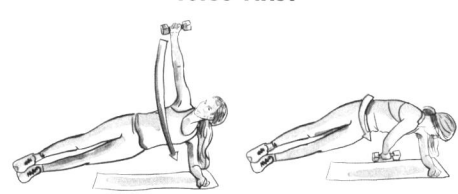

(Left Side) SET 1 REPS: _____ → (Left Side) SET 1 REPS: _____

(Right Side) SET 2 REPS: _____ → (Right Side) SET 2 REPS: _____

(Alternate Sides) SET 3 REPS: _____ → (Alternate Sides) SET 3 REPS: _____

---- 30 SECOND BREAK ----

CIRCUIT 4
30s EACH

4a. Jump Squat

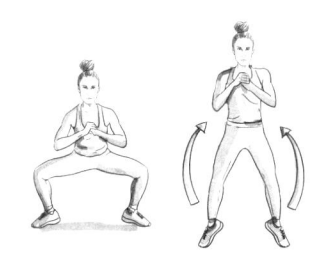

SET 1 REPS: _____ → 15s REST

SET 2 REPS: _____ → 15s REST

SET 3 REPS: _____ → 15s REST

SET 4 REPS: _____ → 15s REST

---- 30 SECOND BREAK ----

COOL DOWN
60s EACH

a. Hamstring Stretch

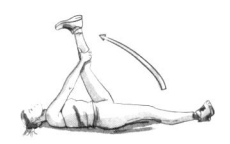

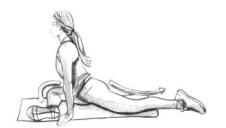

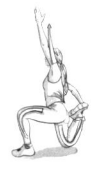

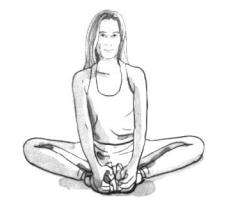

b. Pigeon Stretch

c. Runner's Stretch

d. Butterfly Stretch

TODAY'S WORKOUT INTENSITY: _____ / 10

Workout 35: Resistance Training

DATE _____

1. Bent Over Row

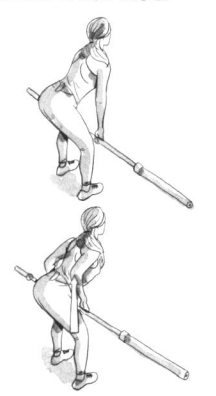

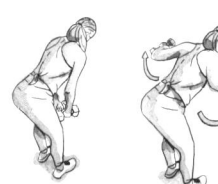

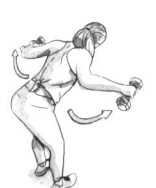

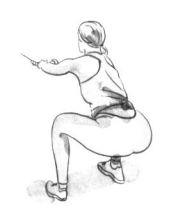

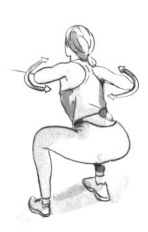

SET 1	REPS: _____	(GOAL: 15-20)	WEIGHT: _____
SET 2	REPS: _____	(GOAL: 12-15)	WEIGHT: _____
SET 3	REPS: _____	(GOAL: 10-12)	WEIGHT: _____
SET 4 (Optional)	REPS: _____	(GOAL: 8-10)	WEIGHT: _____

2. Reverse Dumbbell Fly

SET 1	REPS: _____	(GOAL: 15-20)	WEIGHT: _____
SET 2	REPS: _____	(GOAL: 12-15)	WEIGHT: _____
SET 3	REPS: _____	(GOAL: 10-12)	WEIGHT: _____
SET 4 (Optional)	REPS: _____	(GOAL: 8-10)	WEIGHT: _____

3. Cable Row w/Squat

SET 1	REPS: _____	(GOAL: 15-20)	WEIGHT: _____
SET 2	REPS: _____	(GOAL: 12-15)	WEIGHT: _____
SET 3	REPS: _____	(GOAL: 10-12)	WEIGHT: _____
SET 4 (Optional)	REPS: _____	(GOAL: 8-10)	WEIGHT: _____

4. Deadlift

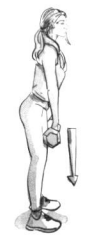

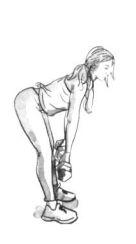

SET 1	REPS: _____	(GOAL: 15-20)	WEIGHT: _____
SET 2	REPS: _____	(GOAL: 12-15)	WEIGHT: _____
SET 3	REPS: _____	(GOAL: 10-12)	WEIGHT: _____
SET 4 (Optional)	REPS: _____	(GOAL: 8-10)	WEIGHT: _____

EXERCISE GUIDE
https://HabitNest.link/booty35

TODAY'S WORKOUT INTENSITY: _____ / 10

EXERCISE GUIDE
https://HabitNest.link/booty36

Workout 36: 4-3-2-1

DATE _____

GLUTE ACTIVATION WARMUP
30s EACH

a. Clam Opener
(30s Each Side)

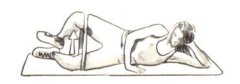

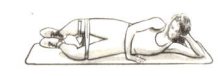

b. Fire Hydrant
(30s Each Side)

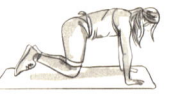

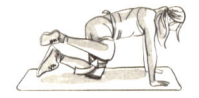

c. Glute Bridge w/ Band Flutter

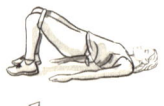

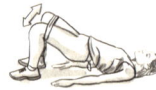

d. Double Walk Out
(2 Steps Right, 2 Steps Left)

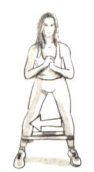

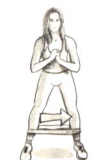

--- 30 SECOND BREAK ---

CIRCUIT 1
60s EACH

1a. Speed Skater
REPS: _____
(Alternate Sides)

→ **1b. Pendulum Lunge**
REPS: _____
(Left Leg)

→ **1c. Pendulum Lunge**
REPS: _____
(Right Leg)

→ **1d. Mountain Climber**
REPS: _____
(Alternate Sides)

--- 30 SECOND BREAK ---

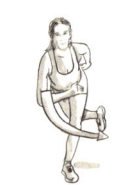

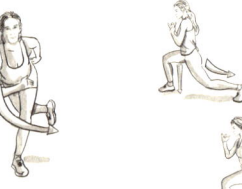

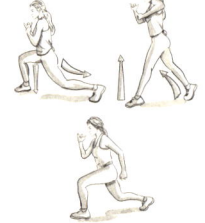

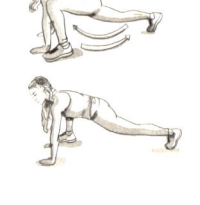

CIRCUIT 2
50s EACH

2a. Plie Squat w/ Shoulder Windmill
SET 1 REPS: _____
SET 2 REPS: _____

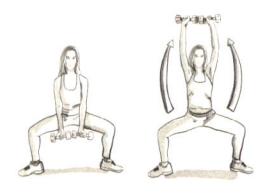

→ **2b. Leap Forward in Squat, Burpee, & Shuffle Back**
SET 1 REPS: _____
SET 2 REPS: _____

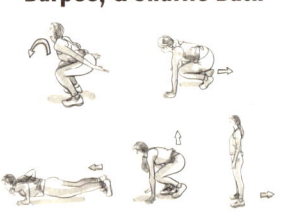

→ **2c. Bulgarian Lunge**
(Left Leg) SET 1 REPS: _____
(Right Leg) SET 2 REPS: _____

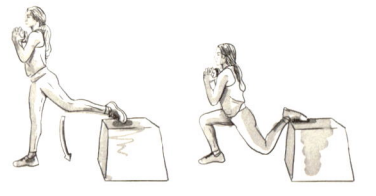

---— 30 SECOND BREAK ———

CIRCUIT 3
(40s EACH)

3a. Vertical Leap

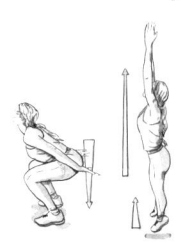

3b. Lateral Lunge w/ Knee to Elbow Rotation

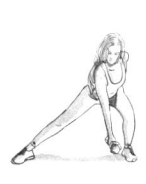

SET 1 REPS: _____ → (Left Leg)   SET 1 REPS: _____

SET 2 REPS: _____ → (Right Leg)   SET 2 REPS: _____

SET 3 REPS: _____ → (Alternate Legs)   SET 3 REPS: _____

———— 30 SECOND BREAK ————

CIRCUIT 4
(30s EACH)

4a. Squat Jack

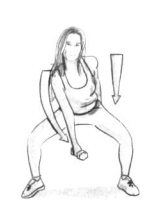

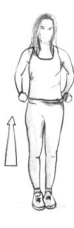

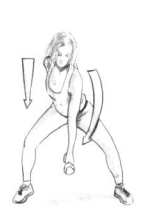

SET 1 REPS: _____ → 15s REST

SET 2 REPS: _____ → 15s REST

SET 3 REPS: _____ → 15s REST

SET 4 REPS: _____ → 15s REST

———— 30 SECOND BREAK ————

COOL DOWN
(60s EACH)

a. Glute Stretch   **b. Pigeon Stretch**   **c. Lat Stretch**   **d. Crossbody Hangover**

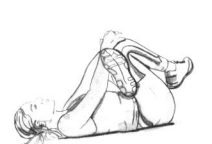

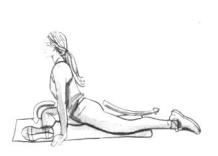

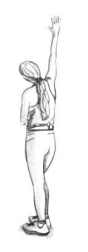

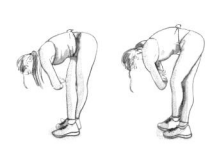

TODAY'S WORKOUT INTENSITY: _____ / 10

EXERCISE GUIDE
https://HabitNest.link/booty37

Workout 37: 4-3-2-1

DATE

GLUTE ACTIVATION WARMUP
30s EACH

a. Clam Opener

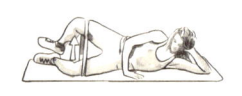

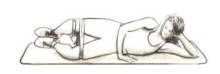

b. Tabletop w/ Donkey Kick

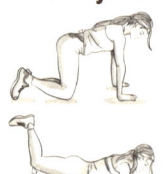

c. Glute Bridge w/ Band Flutter

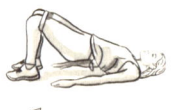

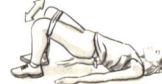

d. Lateral Leg Raise

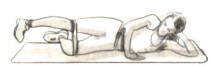

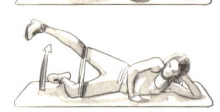

(30s Each Side)

(30s Each Side)

- 30s Each Leg (w/ Foot Flexed)
- 30s Each Leg (w/ Toes Pointing Down)

--- 30 SECOND BREAK ---

CIRCUIT 1
60s EACH

1a. Plank Jack

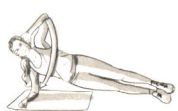

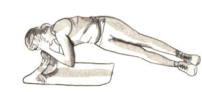

1b. Side Plank w/ Elbow Twist

1c. Side Plank w/ Elbow Twist

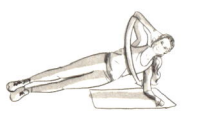

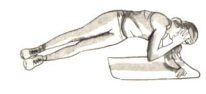

1d. Side Shuffle w/ Floor Tap

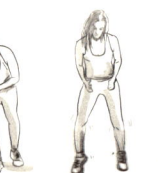

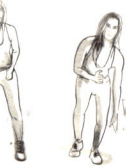

REPS: _____ → REPS: _____ → REPS: _____ → REPS: _____
　　　　　　　　　　　　(Left Side)　　　　　　　(Right Side)

--- 30 SECOND BREAK ---

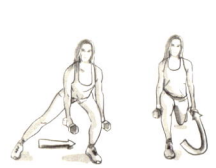

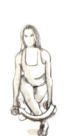

CIRCUIT 2
50s EACH

2a. 3-Point Lunge

2b. Leg Drop

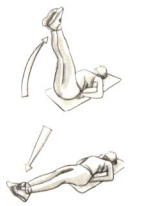

2c. Mountain Climber

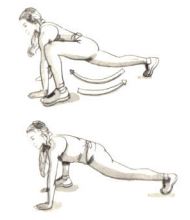

(Left Leg)　SET 1 REPS: _____ → SET 1 REPS: _____ → SET 1 REPS: _____

(Right Leg)　SET 2 REPS: _____ → SET 2 REPS: _____ → SET 2 REPS: _____

--- 30 SECOND BREAK ---

CIRCUIT 3
(40s EACH)

3a. Spider-Man Plank Crunch   3b. Side V-Up

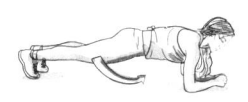

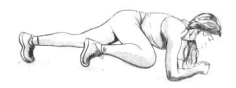

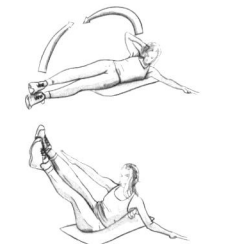

(Alternate Sides) SET 1 REPS: _____ → (Left Side)   SET 1 REPS: _____
(Alternate Sides) SET 2 REPS: _____ → (Right Side)   SET 2 REPS: _____
(Alternate Sides) SET 3 REPS: _____ → (Alternate Sides) SET 3 REPS: _____

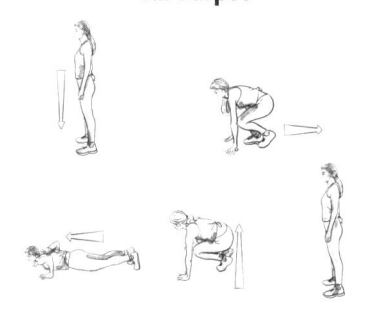

--- 30 SECOND BREAK ---

CIRCUIT 4
(30s EACH)

4a. Burpee

SET 1 REPS: _____ → 15s REST
SET 2 REPS: _____ → 15s REST
SET 3 REPS: _____ → 15s REST
SET 4 REPS: _____ → 15s REST

--- 30 SECOND BREAK ---

COOL DOWN
(60s EACH)

a. Crossbody Hangover   **b. Pigeon Stretch**   **c. Hamstring Stretch**   **d. Runner's Stretch**

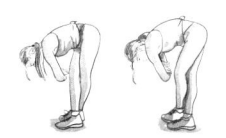

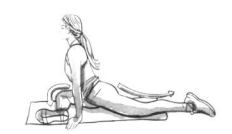

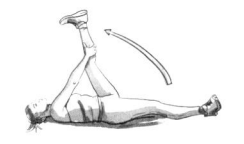

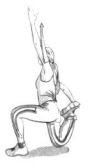

TODAY'S WORKOUT INTENSITY: _____ / 10

Workout 38: Resistance Training

DATE _____

1. Single Leg Glute Bridge

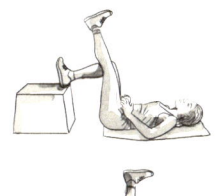

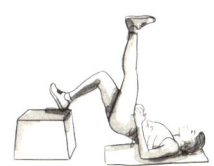

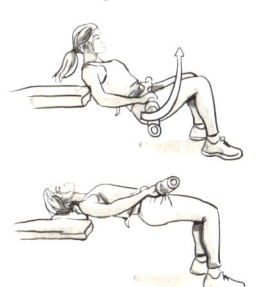

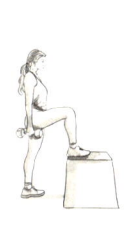

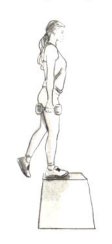

	Left	Right	
SET 1	REPS: _____	(GOAL: 15-20)	WEIGHT: _____
SET 2	REPS: _____	(GOAL: 12-15)	WEIGHT: _____
SET 3	REPS: _____	(GOAL: 10-12)	WEIGHT: _____
SET 4 (Optional)	REPS: _____	(GOAL: 8-10)	WEIGHT: _____

2. Hip Thrust

SET 1	REPS: _____	(GOAL: 15-20)	WEIGHT: _____
SET 2	REPS: _____	(GOAL: 12-15)	WEIGHT: _____
SET 3	REPS: _____	(GOAL: 10-12)	WEIGHT: _____
SET 4 (Optional)	REPS: _____	(GOAL: 8-10)	WEIGHT: _____

3. Alternating Step Up

SET 1	REPS: _____	(GOAL: 15-20)	WEIGHT: _____
SET 2	REPS: _____	(GOAL: 12-15)	WEIGHT: _____
SET 3	REPS: _____	(GOAL: 10-12)	WEIGHT: _____
SET 4 Optional	REPS: _____	(GOAL: 8-10)	WEIGHT: _____

4. Deadlift

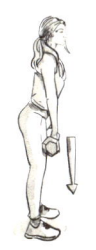

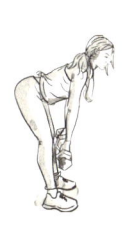

SET 1	REPS: _____	(GOAL: 15-20)	WEIGHT: _____
SET 2	REPS: _____	(GOAL: 12-15)	WEIGHT: _____
SET 3	REPS: _____	(GOAL: 10-12)	WEIGHT: _____
SET 4 (Optional)	REPS: _____	(GOAL: 8-10)	WEIGHT: _____

EXERCISE GUIDE
https://HabitNest.link/booty38

TODAY'S WORKOUT INTENSITY: _____ / 10

Workout 39: 4-3-2-1

EXERCISE GUIDE
https://HabitNest.link/booty39

DATE _____

GLUTE ACTIVATION WARMUP (30s EACH)

a. Clam Opener
(30s Each Side)

b. Box Draw
(Left Side)

c. Box Draw
(Right Side)

d. Running Man
(30s Each Leg)

---30 SECOND BREAK---

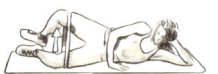

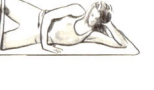

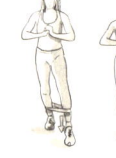

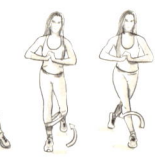

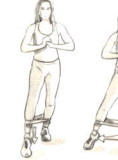

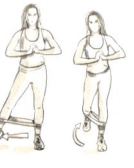

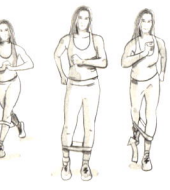

CIRCUIT 1 (60s EACH)

1a. Bulgarian Lunge
REPS: _____ (Left Leg)

1b. Bulgarian Lunge
REPS: _____ (Right Leg)

1c. Jump Twist
REPS: _____

1d. Lateral Lunge
REPS: _____ (Alternate Sides)

---30 SECOND BREAK---

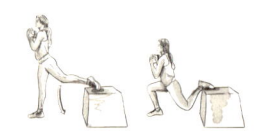

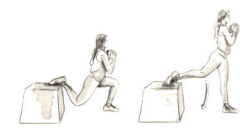

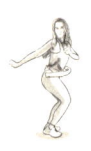

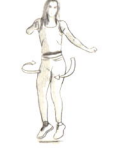

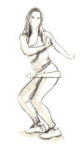

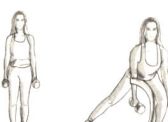

CIRCUIT 2 (50s EACH)

2a. Squat Thrust
SET 1 REPS: _____
SET 2 REPS: _____

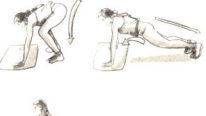

2b. Squat to Overhead Press
SET 1 REPS: _____
SET 2 REPS: _____

2c. The Heisman
SET 1 REPS: _____
SET 2 REPS: _____

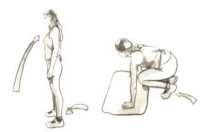

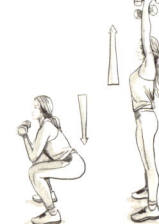

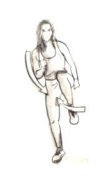

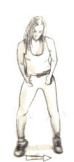

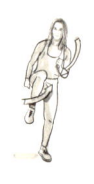

―― 30 SECOND BREAK ――

CIRCUIT 3
40s EACH

3a. Spider-Man Plank Crunch   ### 3b. In and Out Jack

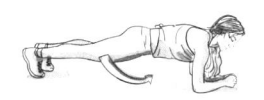

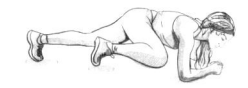

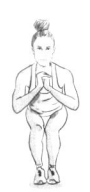

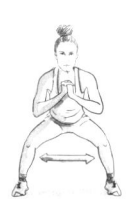

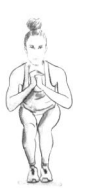

(Alternate Sides) SET 1 REPS: _____ → SET 1 REPS: _____
(Alternate Sides) SET 2 REPS: _____ → SET 2 REPS: _____
(Alternate Sides) SET 3 REPS: _____ → SET 3 REPS: _____

―― 30 SECOND BREAK ――

CIRCUIT 4
30s EACH

4a. Pendulum Jack

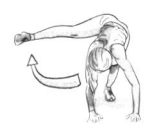

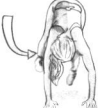

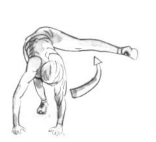

SET 1 REPS: _____ → 15s REST
SET 2 REPS: _____ → 15s REST
SET 3 REPS: _____ → 15s REST
SET 4 REPS: _____ → 15s REST

―― 30 SECOND BREAK ――

COOL DOWN
60s EACH

Hamstring Stretch   **b. Glute Stretch**   **c. Butterfly Stretch**   **d. Pigeon Stretch**

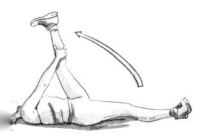

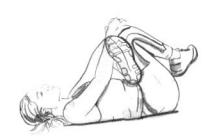

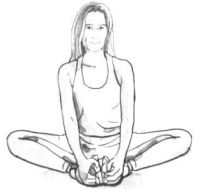

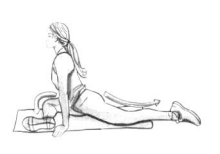

TODAY'S WORKOUT INTENSITY: _____ / 10

Workout 40: Resistance Training

DATE _____

EXERCISE GUIDE
https://HabitNest.link/booty40

1. Lat Pulldown

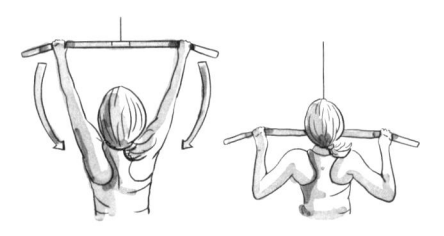

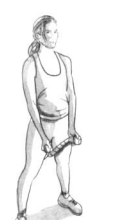

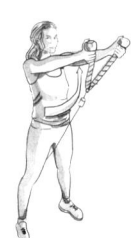

SET 1	REPS: _____ (GOAL: 15-20)	WEIGHT: _____
SET 2	REPS: _____ (GOAL: 12-15)	WEIGHT: _____
SET 3	REPS: _____ (GOAL: 10-12)	WEIGHT: _____
SET 4 (Optional)	REPS: _____ (GOAL: 8-10)	WEIGHT: _____

2. Shoulder Rope Pull

SET 1	REPS: _____ (GOAL: 15-20)	WEIGHT: _____
SET 2	REPS: _____ (GOAL: 12-15)	WEIGHT: _____
SET 3	REPS: _____ (GOAL: 10-12)	WEIGHT: _____
SET 4 (Optional)	REPS: _____ (GOAL: 8-10)	WEIGHT: _____

3. Arnold Press

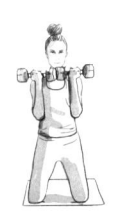

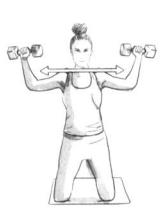

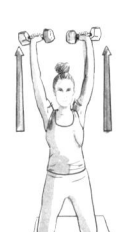

SET 1	REPS: _____ (GOAL: 15-20)	WEIGHT: _____
SET 2	REPS: _____ (GOAL: 12-15)	WEIGHT: _____
SET 3	REPS: _____ (GOAL: 10-12)	WEIGHT: _____
SET 4 (Optional)	REPS: _____ (GOAL: 8-10)	WEIGHT: _____

4. Squat

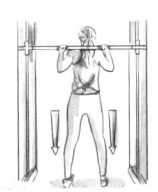

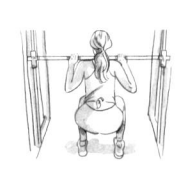

SET 1	REPS: _____ (GOAL: 15-20)	WEIGHT: _____
SET 2	REPS: _____ (GOAL: 12-15)	WEIGHT: _____
SET 3	REPS: _____ (GOAL: 10-12)	WEIGHT: _____
SET 4 (Optional)	REPS: _____ (GOAL: 8-10)	WEIGHT: _____

TODAY'S WORKOUT INTENSITY: _____ / 10

Check-In

How am I ACTUALLY feeling physically?

How am I feeling about the quality and intensity of my workouts? Is my intensity still increasing?

How do I feel about the way I look now compared to when I first started?

What would you like to say to your past self, the one that started this journey?

What would you like to say to future you, who will have an off-day every once in a while?

Bonus Challenge

> *Set a long-term goal to master your eating choices one step at a time.*

You already know that being on top of your nutrition goals will make a significant difference on how your body takes shape. But having perfect nutrition goes way past your body's physical manifestation.

Your daily nutrients are the source of your body's energy. The upside of mastering your nutrition is insane.

Although we built our *Nutrition Sidekick Journal* as a guide for this journey of mastery, it's not a necessity to make major shifts in your eating.

If you are not eating perfectly, there is always a reason - usually multiple. Instead of trying to change all of these eating habits at once (which is incredibly hard and impractical), we invite you to approach the process by **mastering one long-lasting change at a time**.

You may have dozens of little eating habits to change. To list some out:

- *A desire to finish everything on your plate*
- *A feeling that 'food is special / rare' and not to waste rare opportunities to eat specially-prepared food*
- *A feeling that because you ate so well during the week that you deserve to indulge more over the weekend*
- *That if your body is signaling a mood to eat something, the right move is to follow that impulse*

These are all untrue paradigms. Once you realize how to break each of them, your eyes will open to *how much happier* you can be. You will have an utter mastery of food choices and your energy.

You'll be able to walk into ANY situation, any event, and not be ruled by food, which ultimately serves YOU and your body. OWN your food, own your food choices, and you will slowly build your undeniable power over it.

Food mastery is a life-changing skill that will affect you for the rest of your life and serve as your rocket to the land of incredible physique, confidence, health, vitality, and energy.

With one change at a time you will begin to see the momentum, impact, and level of ultimate control you have over your body and your future. Use this fuel to help feed your growth and decision making.

(Optional)
I will commit to being mindful of every food choice I make this week.

_____   _____
Signature   Date

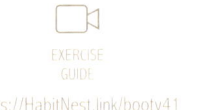

Workout 41: 4-3-2-1

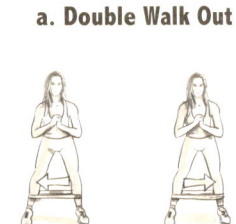

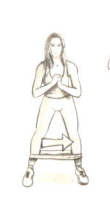

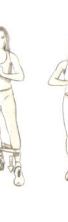

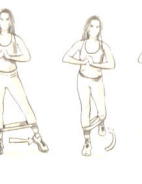

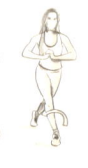

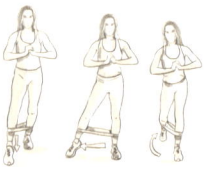

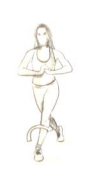

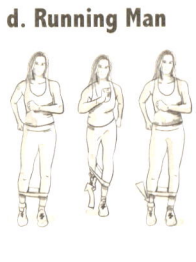

EXERCISE GUIDE
https://HabitNest.link/booty41

DATE _____

GLUTE ACTIVATION WARMUP
(30s EACH)

a. Double Walk Out
(2 Steps Right, 2 Steps Left)

b. Box Draw
(Left Leg)

c. Box Draw
(Right Leg)

d. Running Man
(30s Each Leg)

---

30 SECOND BREAK

CIRCUIT 1
(60s EACH)

1a. Squat Jack
REPS: _____

1b. Plank to Row
REPS: _____
(Alternate Arms)

1c. Plie Squat w/ Shoulder Windmill
REPS: _____

1d. Mountain Climber
REPS: _____
(Alternate Sides)

---

30 SECOND BREAK

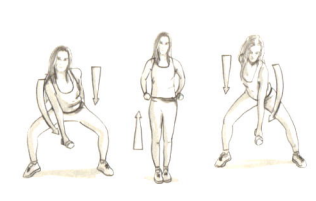

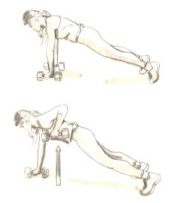

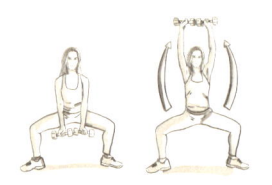

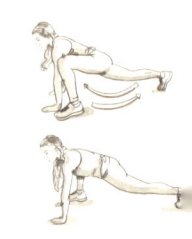

CIRCUIT 2
(50s EACH)

2a. 3-Point Lunge
(Left Leg) SET 1 REPS: _____
(Right Leg) SET 2 REPS: _____

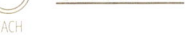

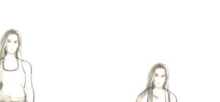

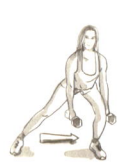

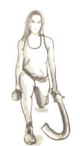

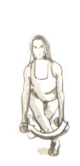

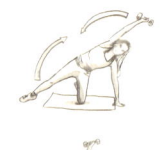

2b. Side Triangle Crunch
(Left Side) SET 1 REPS: _____
(Right Side) SET 2 REPS: _____

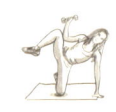

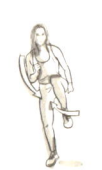

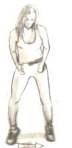

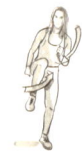

2c. The Heisman
SET 1 REPS: _____
SET 2 REPS: _____

30 SECOND BREAK

CIRCUIT 3

3a. Reverse Dumbbell Fly

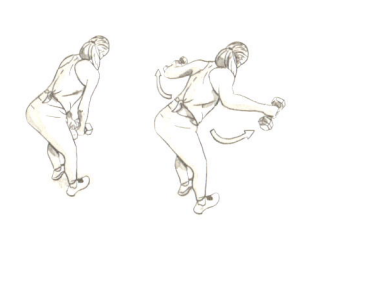

3b. Leap Forward in Squat, Burpee, & Shuffle Back

SET 1 REPS: _____ → SET 1 REPS: _____

SET 2 REPS: _____ → SET 2 REPS: _____

SET 3 REPS: _____ → SET 3 REPS: _____

30 SECOND BREAK

CIRCUIT 4

4a. 4 Donkey Kicks to 4 High Knees

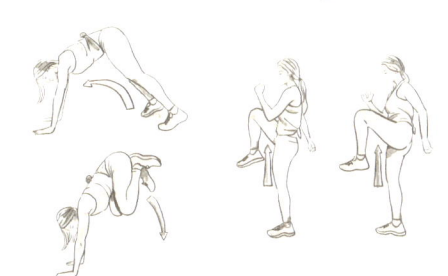

SET 1 REPS: _____ → REST

SET 2 REPS: _____ → REST

SET 3 REPS: _____ → REST

SET 4 REPS: _____ → REST

30 SECOND BREAK

COOL DOWN

a. Pigeon Stretch   **b. Glute Stretch**   **c. Lat Stretch**   **d. Butterfly Stretch**

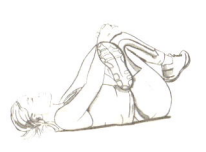

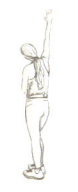

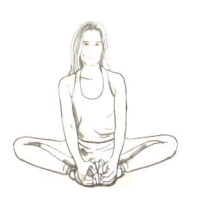

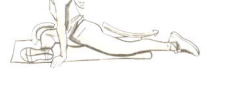

TODAY'S WORKOUT INTENSITY: _____ / 10

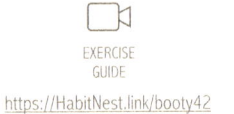

Workout 42: 4-3-2-1

EXERCISE GUIDE
https://HabitNest.link/booty42

DATE _____

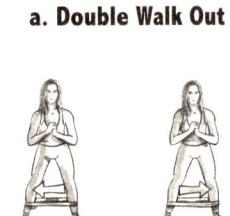

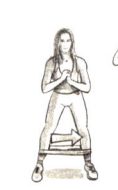

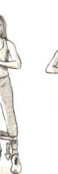

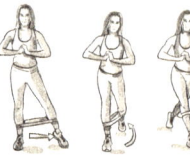

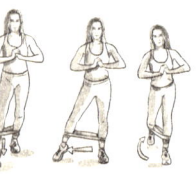

GLUTE ACTIVATION WARMUP (30s EACH)

a. Double Walk Out **b. Box Draw** **c. Box Draw** **d. Running Man**

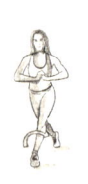

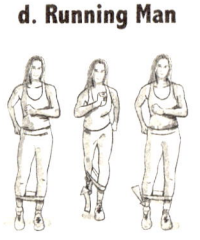

(2 Steps Right, 2 Steps Left) (Left Leg) (Right Leg) (30s Each Leg)

--- 30 SECOND BREAK ---

CIRCUIT 1 (60s EACH)

1a. Burpee **1b. Russian Twist** **1c. Squat to Overhead Press** **1d. Leg Drop**

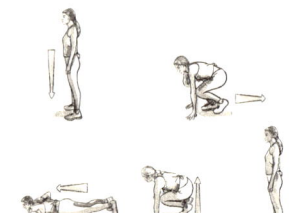

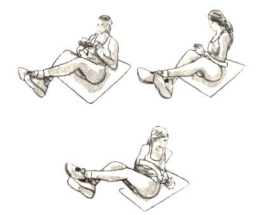

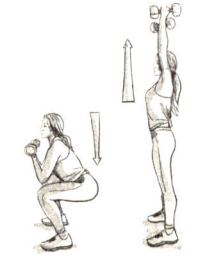

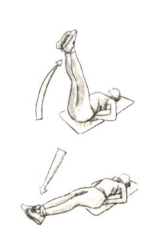

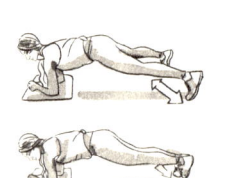

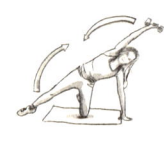

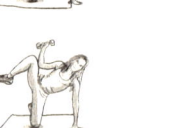

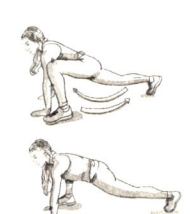

REPS: _____ → REPS: _____ → REPS: _____ → REPS: _____

--- 30 SECOND BREAK ---

CIRCUIT 2 (50s EACH)

2a. Plank Jack **2b. Side Triangle Crunch** **2c. Mountain Climber**

SET 1 REPS: _____ → (Left Side) SET 1 REPS: _____ → SET 1 REPS: _____

SET 2 REPS: _____ → (Right Side) SET 2 REPS: _____ → SET 2 REPS: _____

---------- 30 SECOND BREAK ----------

CIRCUIT 3
40s EACH

3a. Side Plank w/ Torso Rotation

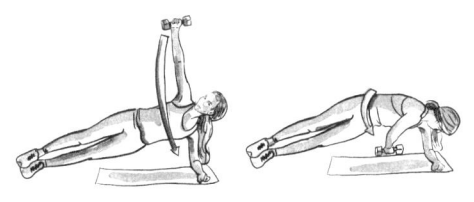

3b. 180° Jump Twist to Floor Tap

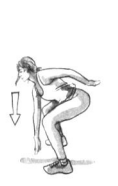

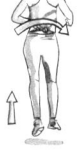

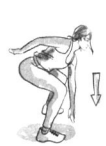

(Left Leg)   SET 1 REPS: _____   →   SET 1 REPS: _____

(Right Leg)   SET 2 REPS: _____   →   SET 2 REPS: _____

(Alternate Legs)   SET t REPS: _____   →   SET 3 REPS: _____

---------- 30 SECOND BREAK ----------

CIRCUIT 4
30s EACH

4a. The Heisman

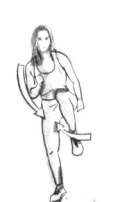

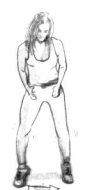

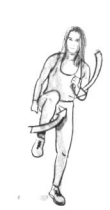

SET 1 REPS: _____   →   15s REST

SET 2 REPS: _____   →   15s REST

SET 3 REPS: _____   →   15s REST

SET 4 REPS: _____   →   15s REST

---------- 30 SECOND BREAK ----------

COOL DOWN
60s EACH

a. Pigeon Stretch   **b. Lat Stretch**   **c. Butterfly Stretch**   **d. Runner's Stretch**

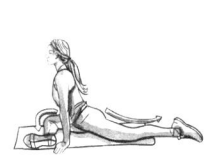

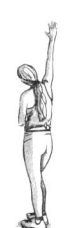

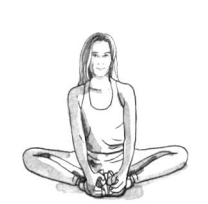

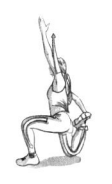

TODAY'S WORKOUT INTENSITY: _____ / 10

Workout 43: Resistance Training

DATE _____

1. Deadlift

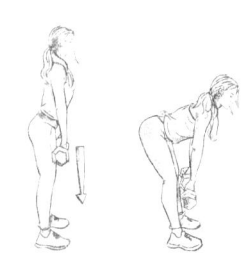

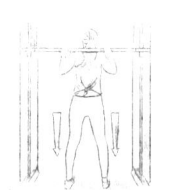

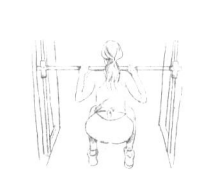

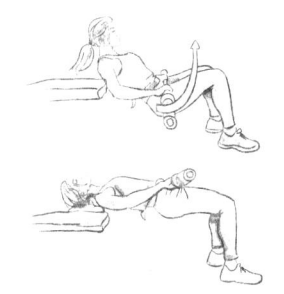

SET 1   REPS: _____   (GOAL: 15-20)   WEIGHT: _____
SET 2   REPS: _____   (GOAL: 12-15)   WEIGHT: _____
SET 3   REPS: _____   (GOAL: 10-12)   WEIGHT: _____
SET 4   REPS: _____   (GOAL: 8-10)   WEIGHT: _____
(Optional)

2. Squat

SET 1   REPS: _____   (GOAL: 15-20)   WEIGHT: _____
SET 2   REPS: _____   (GOAL: 12-15)   WEIGHT: _____
SET 3   REPS: _____   (GOAL: 10-12)   WEIGHT: _____
SET 4   REPS: _____   (GOAL: 8-10)   WEIGHT: _____
(Optional)

3. Hip Thrust

SET 1   REPS: _____   (GOAL: 15-20)   WEIGHT: _____
SET 2   REPS: _____   (GOAL: 12-15)   WEIGHT: _____
SET 3   REPS: _____   (GOAL: 10-12)   WEIGHT: _____
SET 4   REPS: _____   (GOAL: 8-10)   WEIGHT: _____
(Optional)

4. Single Leg Glute Bridge

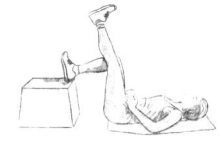

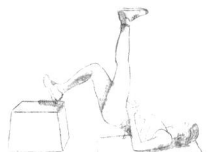

SET 1   REPS: _____   (GOAL: 15-20)   WEIGHT: _____
SET 2   REPS: _____   (GOAL: 12-15)   WEIGHT: _____
SET 3   REPS: _____   (GOAL: 10-12)   WEIGHT: _____
SET 4   REPS: _____   (GOAL: 8-10)   WEIGHT: _____
(Optional)

TODAY'S WORKOUT INTENSITY: _____ / 10

EXERCISE GUIDE
https://HabitNest.link/booty44

Workout 44: 4-3-2-1

DATE

GLUTE ACTIVATION WARMUP
(30s EACH)

a. Double Walk Out
(2 Steps Right, 2 Steps Left)

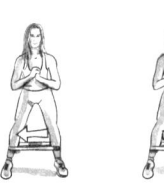

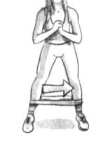

b. Tabletop w/ Donkey Kick
(30s Each Leg)

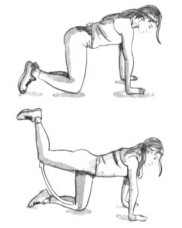

c. Tabletop w/ Diagonal Kick
(30s Each Leg)

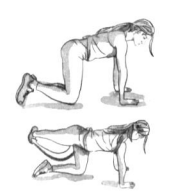

d. Fire Hydrant
(30s Each Leg)

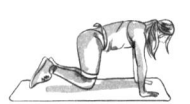

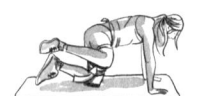

--- 30 SECOND BREAK ---

CIRCUIT 1
(60s EACH)

1a. Ski Mogul

1b. Lateral Lunge w/ Half 'X'

1c. Lateral Lunge w/ Half 'X'

1d. Side Shuffle w/ Floor Tap

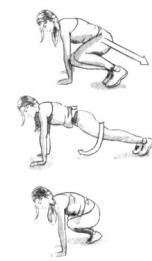

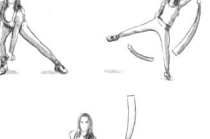

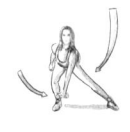

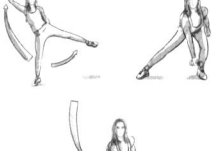

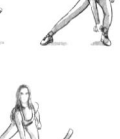

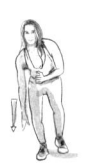

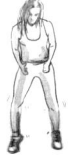

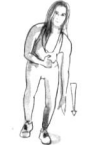

REPS: _____ → REPS: _____ (Left Leg) → REPS: _____ (Right Leg) → REPS: _____

--- 30 SECOND BREAK ---

CIRCUIT 2
(50s EACH)

2a. Squat Thrust

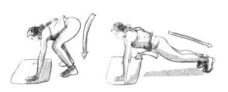

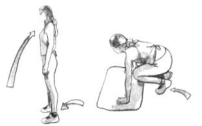

2b. Tabletop Elbow to Knee Crunch

2c. Jump Squat

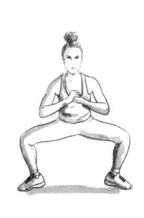

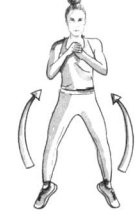

SET 1 REPS: _____ → (Left Side) SET 1 REPS: _____ → SET 1 REPS: _____

SET 2 REPS: _____ → (Right Side) SET 2 REPS: _____ → SET 2 REPS: _____

―――― 30 SECOND BREAK ――――

CIRCUIT 3
(40s EACH)

3a. Lateral Lunge to Curtsy Lunge

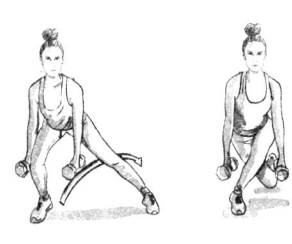

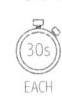

(Left Leg)   SET 1 REPS: _____ →
(Right Leg)   SET 2 REPS: _____ →
(Alternate Legs) SET 3 REPS: _____ →

3b. Side Triangle Crunch

SET 1 REPS: _____
SET 2 REPS: _____
SET 3 REPS: _____

―――― 30 SECOND BREAK ――――

CIRCUIT 4
(30s EACH)

4a. Burpee

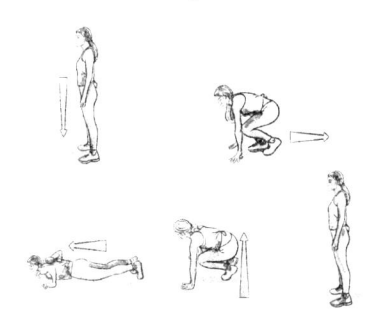

SET 1 REPS: _____ → 15s REST
SET 2 REPS: _____ → 15s REST
SET 3 REPS: _____ → 15s REST
SET 4 REPS: _____ → 15s REST

―――― 30 SECOND BREAK ――――

COOL DOWN
(60s EACH)

a. Crossbody Hangover   **b. Runner's Stretch**   **c. Glute Stretch**   **d. Lat Stretch**

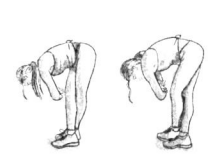

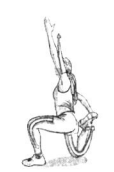

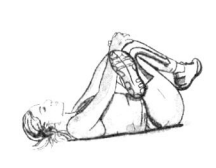

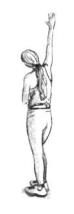

TODAY'S WORKOUT INTENSITY: _____ / 10

Workout 45: Resistance Training

DATE _____

1. Reverse Dumbbell Fly

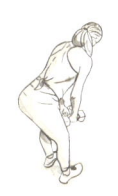

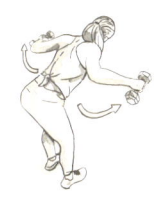

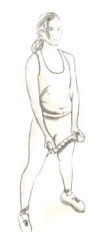

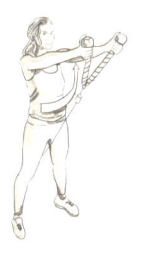

SET 1	REPS: _____	(GOAL: 15-20)	WEIGHT: _____
SET 2	REPS: _____	(GOAL: 12-15)	WEIGHT: _____
SET 3	REPS: _____	(GOAL: 10-12)	WEIGHT: _____
SET 4 (Optional)	REPS: _____	(GOAL: 8-10)	WEIGHT: _____

2. Shoulder Rope Pull

SET 1	REPS: _____	(GOAL: 15-20)	WEIGHT: _____
SET 2	REPS: _____	(GOAL: 12-15)	WEIGHT: _____
SET 3	REPS: _____	(GOAL: 10-12)	WEIGHT: _____
SET 4 (Optional)	REPS: _____	(GOAL: 8-10)	WEIGHT: _____

3. Bent Over Row

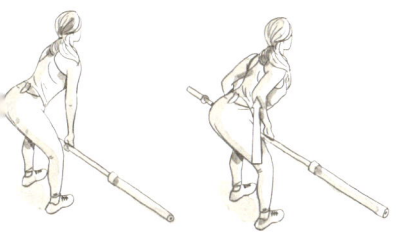

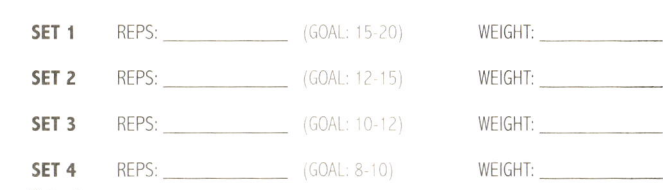

SET 1	REPS: _____	(GOAL: 15-20)	WEIGHT: _____
SET 2	REPS: _____	(GOAL: 12-15)	WEIGHT: _____
SET 3	REPS: _____	(GOAL: 10-12)	WEIGHT: _____
SET 4 (Optional)	REPS: _____	(GOAL: 8-10)	WEIGHT: _____

4. Lateral Raise

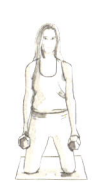

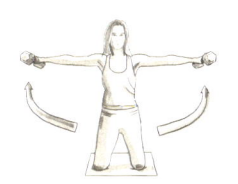

SET 1	REPS: _____	(GOAL: 15-20)	WEIGHT: _____
SET 2	REPS: _____	(GOAL: 12-15)	WEIGHT: _____
SET 3	REPS: _____	(GOAL: 10-12)	WEIGHT: _____
SET 4 (Optional)	REPS: _____	(GOAL: 8-10)	WEIGHT: _____

TODAY'S WORKOUT INTENSITY: _____ / 10

EXERCISE GUIDE
https://HabitNest.link/booty46

Workout 46: 4-3-2-1

DATE _____

GLUTE ACTIVATION WARMUP
(30s EACH)

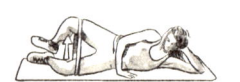

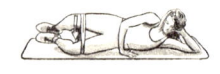

a. Clam Opener
(30s Each Side)

b. Fire Hydrant
(30s Each Side)

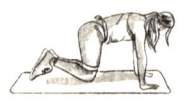

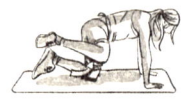

c. Tabletop w/ Donkey Kick
(30s Each Side)

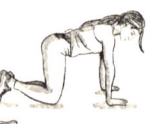

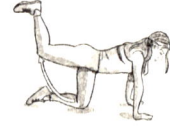

d. Double Walk Out
(2 Steps Right, 2 Steps Left)

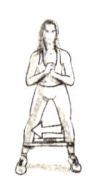

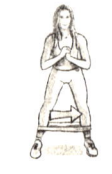

--- 30 SECOND BREAK ---

CIRCUIT 1
(60s EACH)

1a. In and Out Jack
REPS: _____

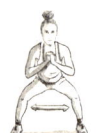

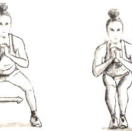

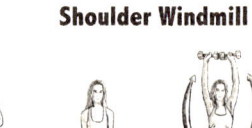

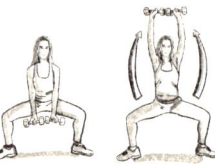

1b. Plie Squat w/ Shoulder Windmill
REPS: _____

1c. High Knee
REPS: _____
(Alternate Sides)

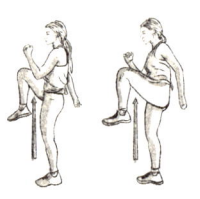

1d. Side to Side Squat
REPS: _____
(Alternate Sides)

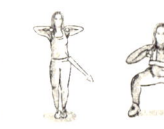

--- 30 SECOND BREAK ---

CIRCUIT 2
(50s EACH)

2a. Speed Skater
SET 1 REPS: _____
SET 2 REPS: _____

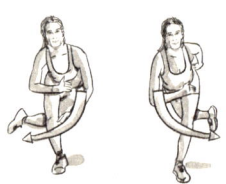

2b. Pendulum Lunge
(Left Leg) SET 1 REPS: _____
(Right Leg) SET 2 REPS: _____

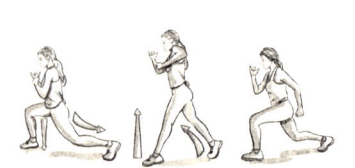

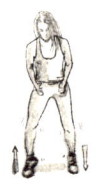

2c. Fast Feet
SET 1 REPS: _____
SET 2 REPS: _____

TODAY'S WORKOUT INTENSITY: _____ / 10

---
30 SECOND BREAK

CIRCUIT 3
(40s EACH)

3a. Lateral Lunge to Curtsy Lunge

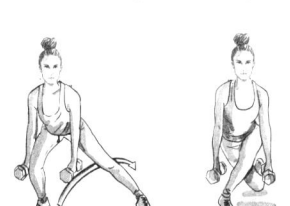

3b. Boxing Jab

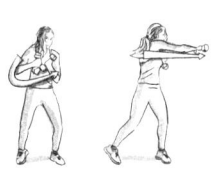

(Left Leg)   SET 1 REPS: _____   →   SET 1 REPS: _____

(Right Leg)   SET 2 REPS: _____   →   SET 2 REPS: _____

(Alternate Legs) SET 3 REPS: _____   →   SET 3 REPS: _____

---
30 SECOND BREAK

CIRCUIT 4
(30s EACH)

4a. Burpee

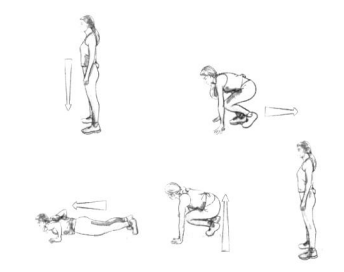

SET 1 REPS: _____   →   15s REST

SET 2 REPS: _____   →   15s REST

SET 3 REPS: _____   →   15s REST

SET 4 REPS: _____   →   15s REST

---
30 SECOND BREAK

COOL DOWN
(60s EACH)

a. Hamstring Stretch   **b. Glute Stretch**   **c. Butterfly Stretch**   **d. Runner's Stretch**

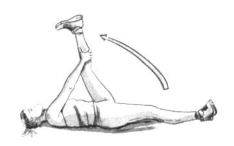

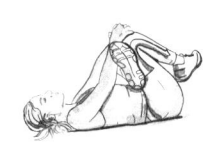

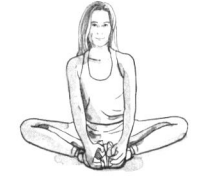

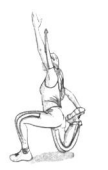

TODAY'S WORKOUT INTENSITY: _____ / 10

Workout 47: 4-3-2-1

EXERCISE GUIDE
https://HabitNest.link/booty47

DATE _____

GLUTE ACTIVATION WARMUP
30s EACH

a. Clam Opener   **b. Tabletop w/ Donkey Kick**   **c. Fire Hydrant**   **d. Lateral Leg Raise**

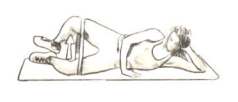

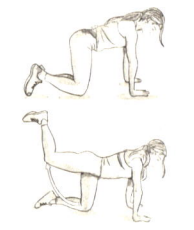

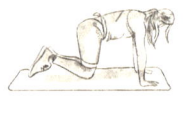

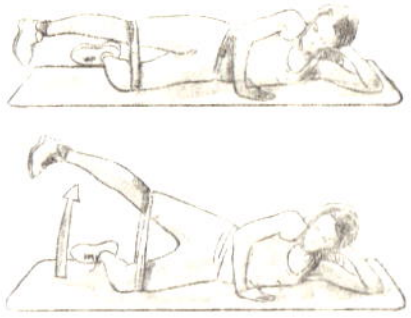

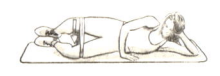

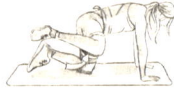

(30s Each Side)   (30s Each Side)   (30s Each Side)   - 30s Each Leg w/ Foot Flexed
     - 30s Each Leg w/ Toes Pointing Down

--- 30 SECOND BREAK ---

CIRCUIT 1
60s EACH

1a. Plank Step Up   **1b. Vertical Leap**   **1c. Side Triangle Crunch**   **1d. Side Triangle Crunch**

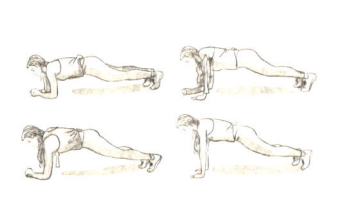

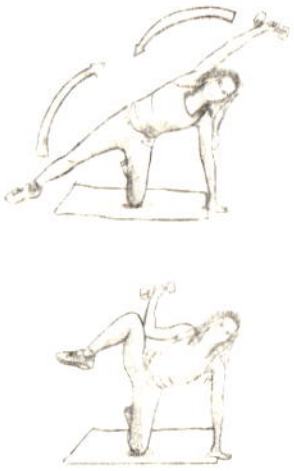

REPS: _____ → REPS: _____ → REPS: _____ → REPS: _____
(Alternate Arms)   (Left Side)   (Right Side)

--- 30 SECOND BREAK ---

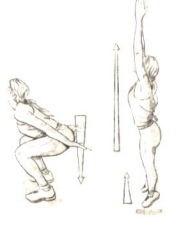

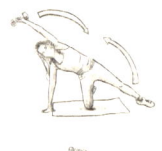

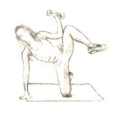

CIRCUIT 2
50s EACH

2a. Squat Thrust   **2b. V-Up**   **2c. Roundhouse Kick to Squat**

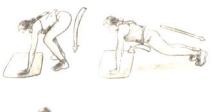

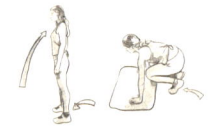

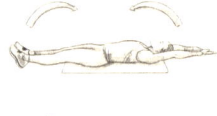

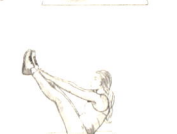

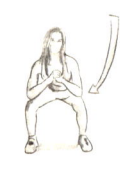

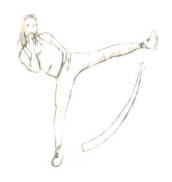

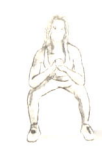

SET 1 REPS: _____ → SET 1 REPS: _____ → (Left Leg) SET 1 REPS: _____

SET 2 REPS: _____ → SET 2 REPS: _____ → (Right Leg) SET 2 REPS: _____

---------- 30 SECOND BREAK ----------

CIRCUIT 3
(40s EACH)

3a. Lateral Lunge to Curtsy Lunge

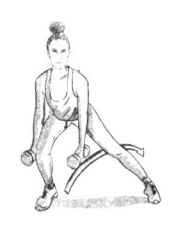

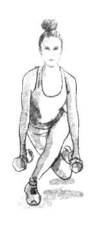

3b. Mountain Climber

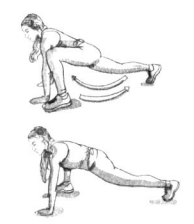

(Left Leg)	SET 1 REPS: _____	→	SET 1 REPS: _____
(Right Leg)	SET 2 REPS: _____	→	SET 2 REPS: _____
(Alternate Legs)	SET 3 REPS: _____	→	SET 3 REPS: _____

---------- 30 SECOND BREAK ----------

CIRCUIT 4
(30s EACH)

4a. Burpee

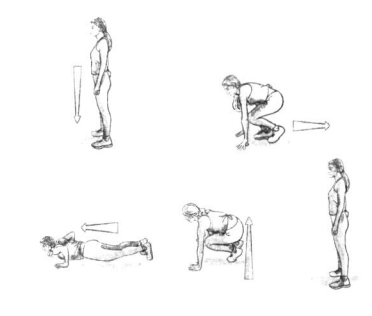

SET 1 REPS: _____ → 15s REST
SET 2 REPS: _____ → 15s REST
SET 3 REPS: _____ → 15s REST
SET 4 REPS: _____ → 15s REST

---------- 30 SECOND BREAK ----------

COOL DOWN
(60s EACH)

a. Hamstring Stretch   **b. Crossbody Hangover**   **c. Pigeon Stretch**   **d. Butterfly Stretch**

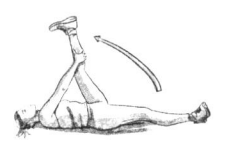

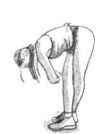

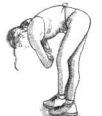

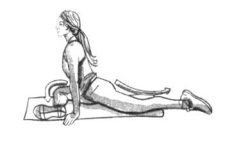

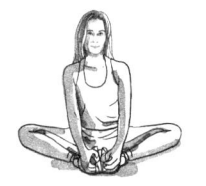

TODAY'S WORKOUT INTENSITY: _____ / 10

Workout 48: Resistance Training

DATE _____

1. Single Leg Glute Bridge

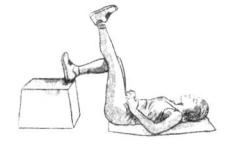

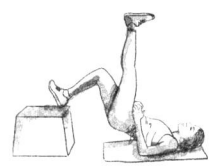

                                  <u>Left</u>   <u>Right</u>

SET 1   REPS: _____   (GOAL: 15-20)   WEIGHT: _____

SET 2   REPS: _____   (GOAL: 12-15)   WEIGHT: _____

SET 3   REPS: _____   (GOAL: 10-12)   WEIGHT: _____

SET 4   REPS: _____   (GOAL: 8-10)   WEIGHT: _____
(Optional)

2. Hip Thrust

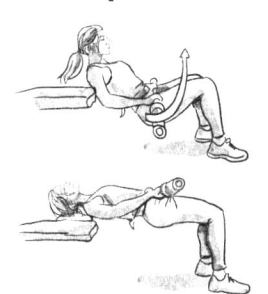

SET 1   REPS: _____   (GOAL: 15-20)   WEIGHT: _____

SET 2   REPS: _____   (GOAL: 12-15)   WEIGHT: _____

SET 3   RFPS: _____   (GOAL: 10-12)   WEIGHT: _____

SET 4   REPS: _____   (GOAL: 8-10)   WEIGHT: _____
(Optional)

3. Single Leg Deadlift

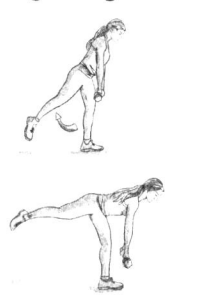

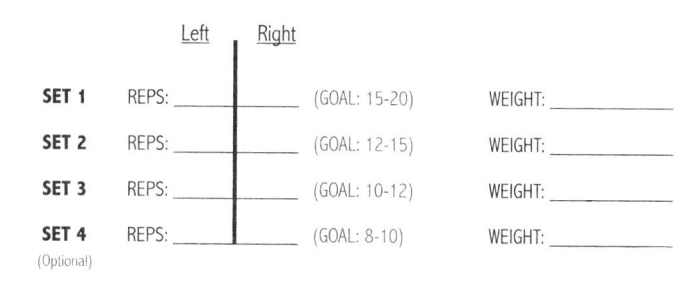

                                  <u>Left</u>   <u>Right</u>

SET 1   REPS: _____   (GOAL: 15-20)   WEIGHT: _____

SET 2   REPS: _____   (GOAL: 12-15)   WEIGHT: _____

SET 3   REPS: _____   (GOAL: 10-12)   WEIGHT: _____

SET 4   REPS: _____   (GOAL: 8-10)   WEIGHT: _____
(Optional)

4. Squat

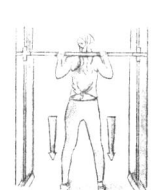

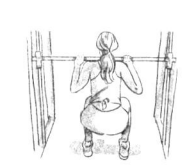

SET 1   REPS: _____   (GOAL: 15-20)   WEIGHT: _____

SET 2   REPS: _____   (GOAL: 12-15)   WEIGHT: _____

SET 3   REPS: _____   (GOAL: 10-12)   WEIGHT: _____

SET 4   REPS: _____   (GOAL: 8-10)   WEIGHT: _____
(Optional)

TODAY'S WORKOUT INTENSITY: _____ / 10

EXERCISE GUIDE
https://HabitNest.link/booty49

Workout 49: 4-3-2-1

DATE _____

GLUTE ACTIVATION WARMUP
30s EACH

a. Double Walk Out
(2 Steps Right, 2 Steps Left)

b. Box Draw
(Left Leg)

c. Box Draw
(Right Leg)

d. Running Man
(30s Each Leg)

---- 30 SECOND BREAK ----

CIRCUIT 1
60s EACH

1a. In and Out Jack

1b. Plank to Row

1c. Mountain Climber

1d. Starfish Crunch

REPS: _____ → REPS: _____ (Alternate Arms) → REPS: _____ (Alternate Sides) → REPS: _____ (Alternate Sides)

---- 30 SECOND BREAK ----

CIRCUIT 2
50s EACH

2a. Roundhouse Kick to Squat

2b. Side Plank w/ Torso Rotation

2c. The Heisman

(Left Leg) SET 1 REPS: _____ → (Left Side) SET 1 REPS: _____ → SET 1 REPS: _____

(Right Leg) SET 2 REPS: _____ → (Right Side) SET 2 REPS: _____ → SET 2 REPS: _____

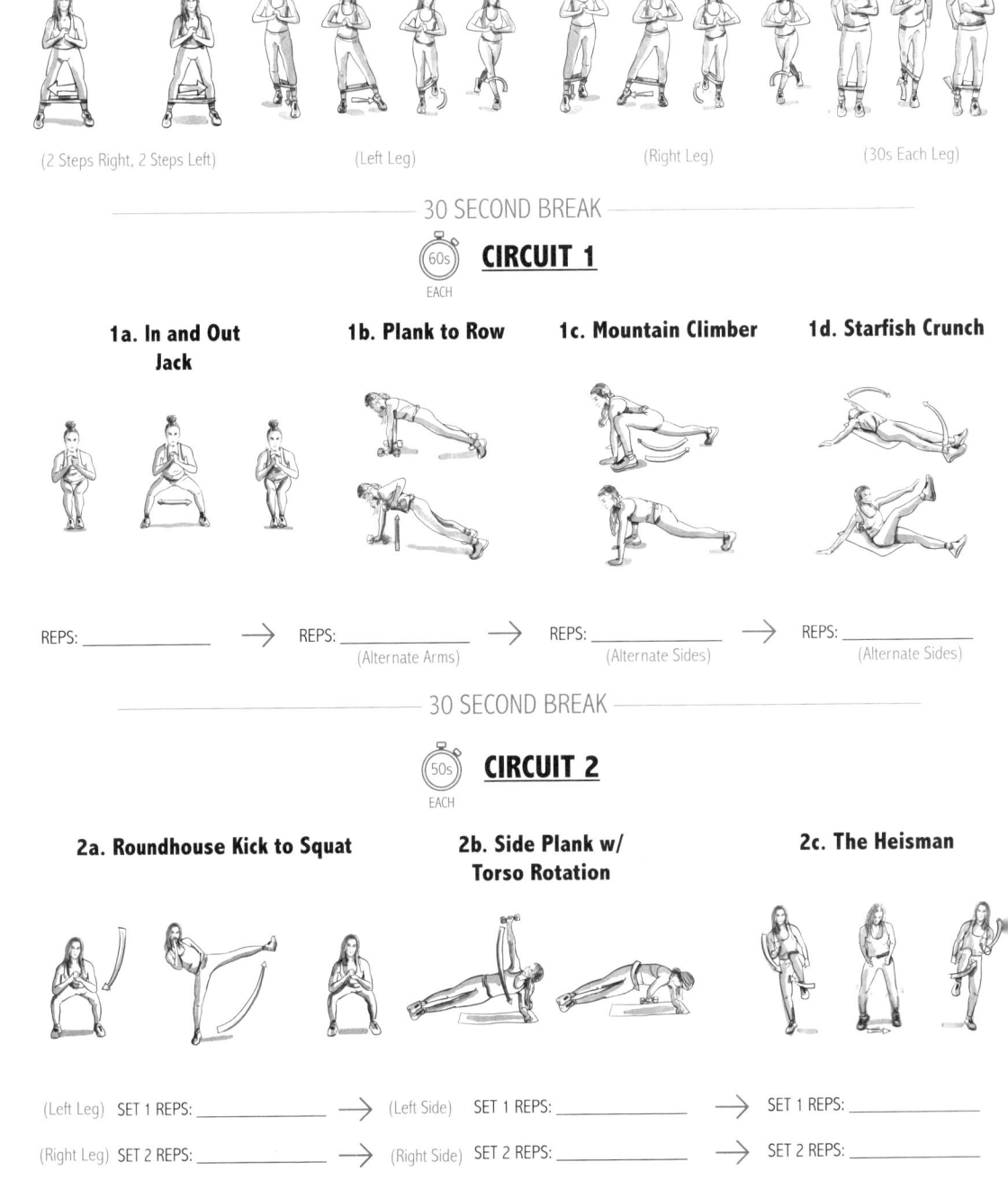

--- 30 SECOND BREAK ---

CIRCUIT 3
40s EACH

3a. Plie Jump Squat

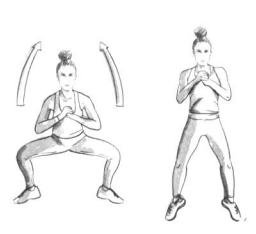

SET 1 REPS: _____
SET 2 REPS: _____
SET 3 REPS: _____

→ (Left Side)
→ (Right Side)
→ (Alternating Sides)

3b. Standing Side Crunch

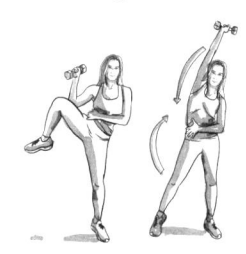

SET 1 REPS: _____
SET 2 REPS: _____
SET 3 REPS: _____

--- 30 SECOND BREAK ---

CIRCUIT 4
30s EACH

4a. Leap Forward in Squat, Burpee, & Shuffle Back

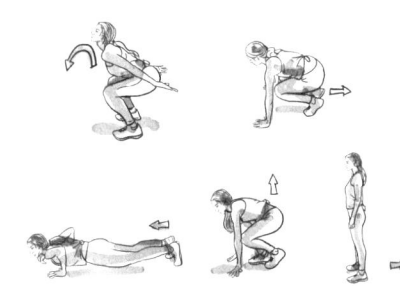

SET 1 REPS: _____ → 15s REST
SET 2 REPS: _____ → 15s REST
SET 3 REPS: _____ → 15s REST
SET 4 REPS: _____ → 15s REST

--- 30 SECOND BREAK ---

COOL DOWN
60s EACH

a. Pigeon Stretch **b. Runner's Stretch** **c. Glute Stretch** **d. Lat Stretch**

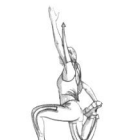

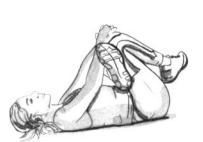

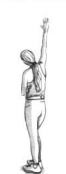

Workout 50: Resistance Training

DATE _____

1. Squat

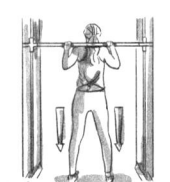

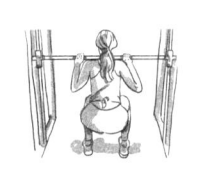

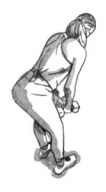

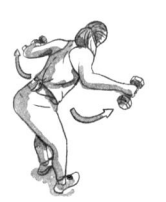

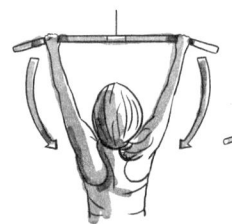

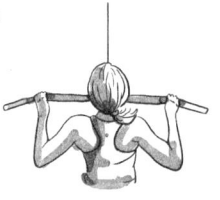

SET 1	REPS: _____ (GOAL: 15-20)	WEIGHT: _____
SET 2	REPS: _____ (GOAL: 12-15)	WEIGHT: _____
SET 3	REPS: _____ (GOAL: 10-12)	WEIGHT: _____
SET 4 (Optional)	REPS: _____ (GOAL: 8-10)	WEIGHT: _____

2. Reverse Dumbbell Fly

SET 1	REPS: _____ (GOAL: 15-20)	WEIGHT: _____
SET 2	REPS: _____ (GOAL: 12-15)	WEIGHT: _____
SET 3	REPS: _____ (GOAL: 10-12)	WEIGHT: _____
SET 4 (Optional)	REPS: _____ (GOAL: 8-10)	WEIGHT: _____

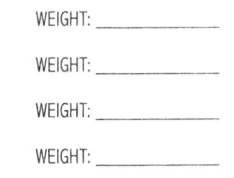

3. Lat Pulldown

SET 1	REPS: _____ (GOAL: 15-20)	WEIGHT: _____
SET 2	REPS: _____ (GOAL: 12-15)	WEIGHT: _____
SET 3	REPS: _____ (GOAL: 10-12)	WEIGHT: _____
SET 4 (Optional)	REPS: _____ (GOAL: 8-10)	WEIGHT: _____

4. Lateral Raise

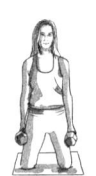

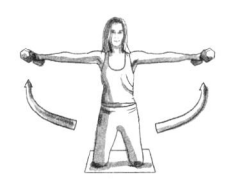

SET 1	REPS: _____ (GOAL: 15-20)	WEIGHT: _____
SET 2	REPS: _____ (GOAL: 12-15)	WEIGHT: _____
SET 3	REPS: _____ (GOAL: 10-12)	WEIGHT: _____
SET 4 (Optional)	REPS: _____ (GOAL: 8-10)	WEIGHT: _____

EXERCISE GUIDE
https://HabitNest.link/booty50

TODAY'S WORKOUT INTENSITY: _____ / 10

<u>Congratulations!!!</u>

You've made it to the end of the journal and completed an INTENSE interval training & weightlifting regimen that has no doubt increased your strength, appearance, confidence, and ability to accomplish your goals.

For you to have gotten this far means you've earned a very serious congratulations. You need to celebrate because your willpower and confidence should be soaring through the roof.

You've gained lessons about yourself not many dare to approach. You've struggled with your own mind, body and heart and gained some serious control over them. You fully understand that you have the power in you to accomplish ANY goal you put your mind to.

That's so awesome.

You are a true WARRIOR.

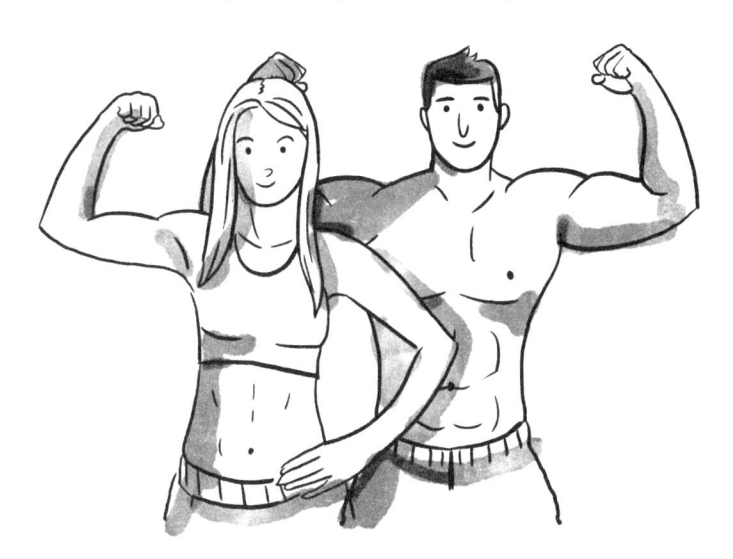

We LOVE sharing stories of our users and what their lives looked like BEFORE using the journal compared to where they are NOW!

If you want to share your story with us, you can do so here: habitnest.com/badasstestimonial

Check-In

How has my life changed since I started this program?

_____
_____
_____
_____

What changes have I seen in my attitude?

_____
_____
_____
_____

What physical changes have I seen?

_____
_____
_____
_____

How do I feel about myself in general compared to when I started this program?

_____
_____
_____
_____

How do I see myself continuing to build on what I've learned and gained by doing this program?

_____
_____
_____
_____

- Fin -

So... What Now?

So you've gotten through the program, seen incredible results, learned that you have immense strength in you to accomplish your goals, and hopefully you're more confident than ever!

Although you should feel very accomplished for getting through this entire program... know that you started the program to continually improve your life. *Don't stop now. This is only the beginning.*

Remember: **Every single day in your life where you take the time to work towards a more physically energized, fitter, confident version of yourself will automatically be a better day in your life.**

You only stand to gain from continuing work towards your fitness goals.

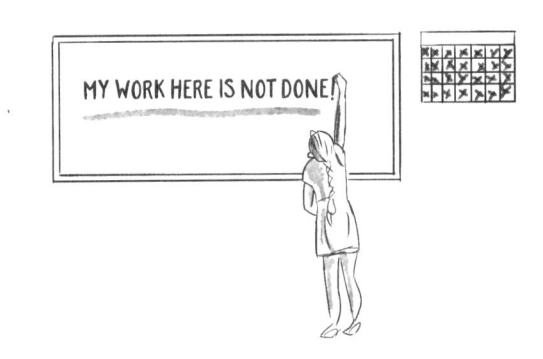

Shop Habit Nest Products

Lifestyle Products

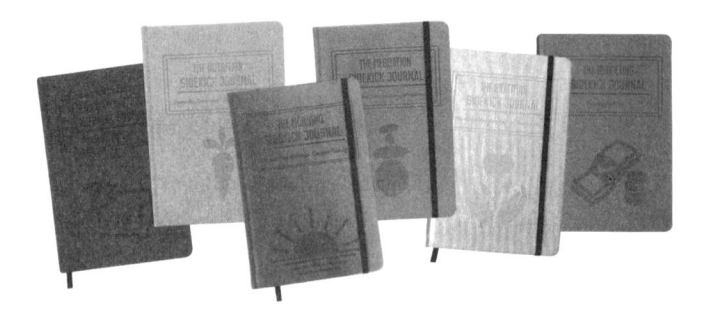

All of our lifestyle journals come with **daily content** (including Pro-Tips, Daily Challenges, Practical Resources, & more) to inspire you and give you bite-sized information to use along your journey. They also contain **daily questions aimed at holding you accountable** to ingraining that habit into your life.

The Morning Sidekick Journal Series

A set of guided morning planners that help you conquer your mornings and conquer your life. This complete 4-volume series covers one year of morning routines.

The Evening Routine & Sleep Sidekick Journal

Helps you to wind down your days peacefully, prepare for each next day, and get the most rejuvenating sleep of your life.

The Gratitude Sidekick Journal Series

A set of research-based journals that will help make an attitude of appreciation
a core part of who you are. There are 3 Volumes in total.

The Meditation Sidekick Journal

Built to give you all the tools you need to stay consistent with a meditation practice.

The Nutrition Sidekick Journal

Your nutrition tracker, informational guide, and coach, all in one.

The Budgeting Sidekick Journal Series

The most simple-yet-effective budgeting guide in the world, helping you find full clarity on your budgeting goals and to achieve financial freedom. Set spending goals, track your daily spending, and reconcile along the way. Contains two volumes, which cover well over a year of budgeting.

Fitness Products

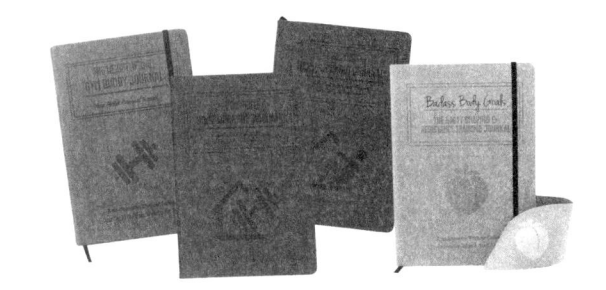

Our no-nonsense fitness books have fully guided fitness routines. No thinking required; just open the books and follow along.

The Weightlifting Gym Buddy Journal Series

A set of guided personal training programs aimed at helping you have the best workouts of your life. This complete 4-volume series covers one year of weightlifting workouts.

The Bodyweight / Dumbbell Home Workout Journals

Specifically focus on HOME workout programs that require minimal-to-no equipment to complete.

The Badass Body Goals Journal

An at-home-friendly fitness journal that focuses on HIIT and circuit workouts.
This journal comes with a full video guide you can play and follow along.

Other Products

The Habit Nest Daily Planner

Plan your day including your top priorities, smaller 5-minute tasks, and all your to-dos. Get optional suggestions for ways to start your mornings and end your evenings with as well.

George The Short-Necked Giraffe (Children's Book)

Follow along George's journey as he learns the hard way that fully accepting himself, exactly the way he is, is the only path to living his happiest life.

Shop all products here: **habitnest.com/store**

The Habit Nest Mobile App

The Habit Nest app offers a **digital representation of our journals**, with the benefit of improved tracking, varying ways to showcase content, and gamification, and more.

When Habit Nest was initially founded, it was supposed to be in mobile app form from the start.

As a team of three young founders with no outside funding to get a mobile app built, we started with paper journals that worked using the same concept,
which you're currently holding.

5 years and hundreds of thousands of journals sold later, we were finally able to create our mobile app and released it at the end of 2021.

We will always continue to print physical journals for every habit we release, only now, they'll also be put into the app so that everyone can experience our habit journeys in the way that suits them best.

If you're interested in seeing seeing whether the app is right for you, feel free to see more at **habitnest.com/app**

With a lot of love,

Mikey Ahdoot, Ari Banayan, & Amir Atighehchi
Co-Founders of Habit Nest

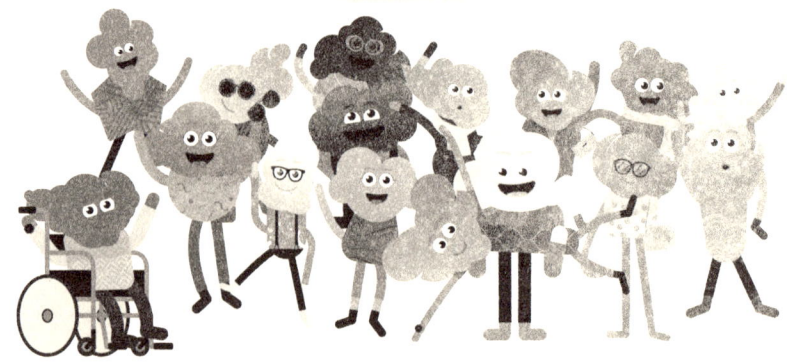

The Phoenixes Access Pass

We released *The Phoenixes* - Habit Nest's Special Access Pass - in 2022.

Anyone who purchases a Phoenix gets:

1. **Lifetime access** to the Habit Nest app.
2. Access to a **Learn2Earn system** we're building within the app, in which you will have chances to earn prizes/rewards for using our app to build better habits.
3. **First dibs** on new journal releases & our best discounts.

If you're interested in purchasing a Phoenix, visit:
https://habitnest.com/vip

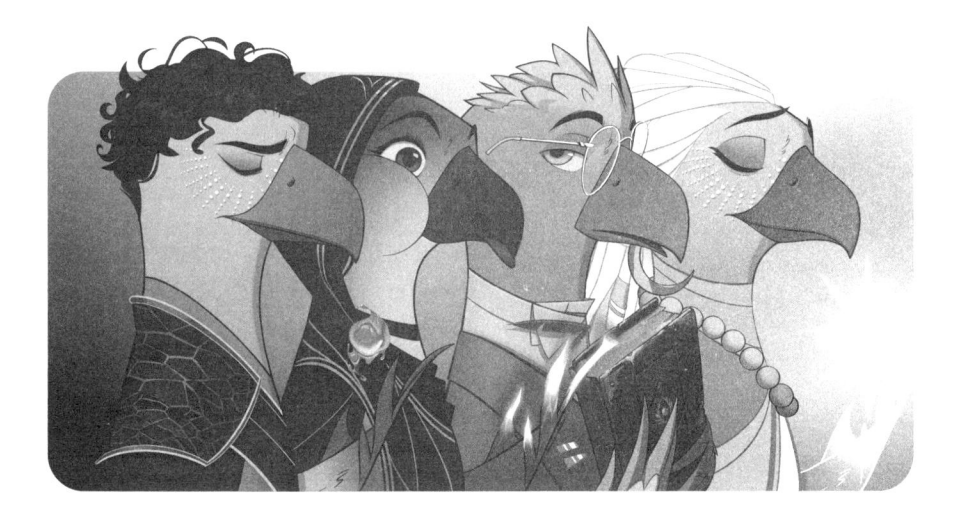

For more information, follow The Phoenixes on Twitter: **@thephoenixesnft**

Workout Index

Workout Index

1. *Glute Activation Warmups*
2. *4-3-2-1 Exercises*
3. *Resistance Training Exercises*
4. *Stretches*

Glute Activation Warmups

4 Donkey Kicks to 4 High Knees

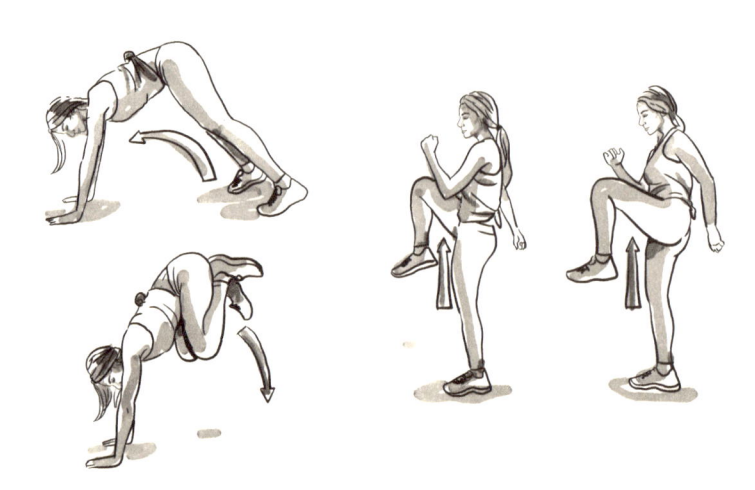

1. Start in a downward dog position with your arms and feet shoulder-width apart.

2. Kick your feet and calves upwards towards your tailbone while bracing your core and shifting your weight to your arms.

3. Repeat this three more times.

4. Stand straight up with your feet shoulder-width apart.

5. Run in place 4 times while raising your knees as high as possible as you alternate legs.

6. Repeat until the set is complete!

Glute Activation Warmups

Box Draw

1. Wrap the resistance band around your calves or ankles.

2. Get into a squat position with your knees bent and your feet shoulder-width apart.

3. Staying low in squat position, take a step forward, then to the right, then behind you, and then diagonally behind you all with the same leg.

4. Keep your core tight and your glute muscles squeezed as you complete the exercise.

5. Repeat.

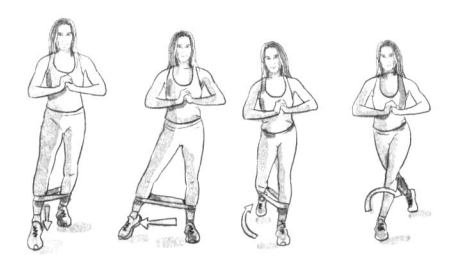

Burpee

1. Stand straight up.

2. Bring both hands towards the floor, and once they're on the floor, extend both legs so they're straight behind you.

3. Jump or step your feet back to your hands.

4. Using your arms for momentum, jump up as high as you can while reaching your hands towards the ceiling.

6. Repeat until the set is complete!

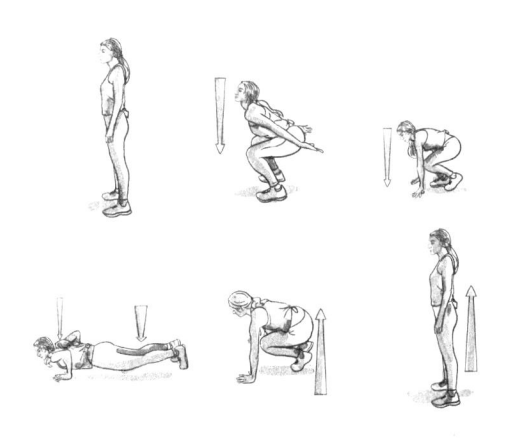

Glute Activation Warmups

Clam Opener

1. Wrap the resistance band just over your knees

2. Lie on your leg side with your knees bent and your feet together.

3. Open your knees apart as widely as possible while squeezing the glute muscles in your right leg as tightly as possible.

4. Slowly allow the knee to come down so that they're together again on the floor, and repeat the movement.

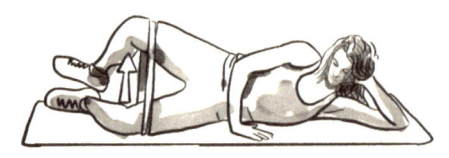

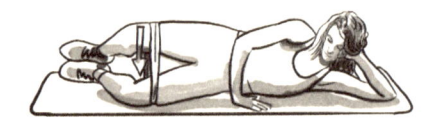

Double Walk Out

1. Wrap the resistance bands around your calves or ankles.

2. Get into a squat position with your knees slightly bent and your feet shoulder-width apart.

3. Staying low in squat position, take a step to the right while maintaining the low squat position.

4. Step back to the original position, starting with your left leg.

5. Repeat.

*The double side step is the same movement, except you take two steps to the side and then return.

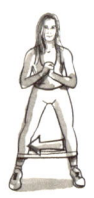

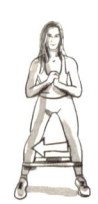

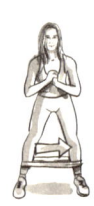

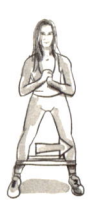

Glute Activation Warmups

Fire Hydrant

1. Wrap a resistance band around your thighs just above your knees.
2. Get into a Table-Top position with your knees and hands on the floor.
3. Keeping your knee bent, raise one leg laterally off the floor.
4. Repeat this until the set is complete.

Note: You can do this with or without the resistance band.

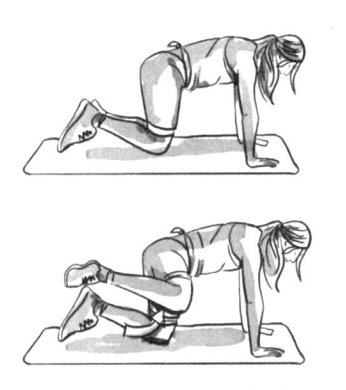

Glute Bridge w/Band Flutter

1. Lift your hips off the ground while keeping your toes pointed forward.

2. Open and close your knees together. When closing your knees, leave some tension in the band (don't close your legs all the way so the band doesn't get loose).

3. Try to keep your hips as centered as possible without dipping from side to side. Don't let your hips drop.

Note: Try and keep your hips as high as possible while doing this move.

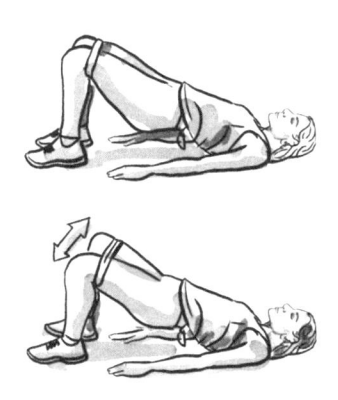

Glute Activation Warmups

Glute Bridge w/Leg Extension

1. Lift your hips off the ground while keeping your toes pointed forward.

2. From here, extend one leg while squeezing your glutes. If you alternate legs, make sure to keep your glutes squeezed.

3. Try to keep your hips as centered as possible without dipping from side to side. Don't let your hips drop.

Note: Try and keep your hips as high as possible while doing this move. Lateral Leg Raise w/ Flexed Foot.

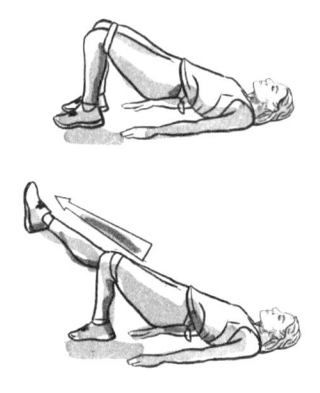

Lateral Leg Raise w/Foot Flexed

1. Lie on your side with your head resting in your hand.

2. From here, lift your leg up while keeping your foot flexed.

3. When returning your foot to the starting position, make sure to leave tension in the band (don't come low enough with your leg that the band becomes loose).

4. Repeat the movement while making sure your foot stays flexed.

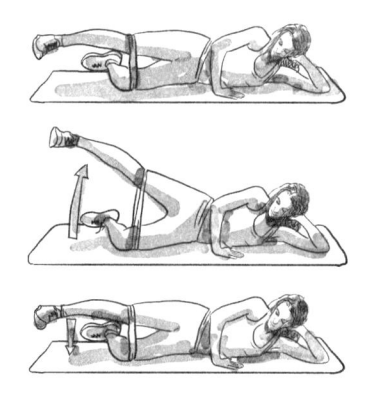

Glute Activation Warmups

Lateral Leg Raise w/ Toes Pointing Down

1. Lie on your side with your head resting in your hand.

2. From here, lift your leg up while keeping your foot and toes pointed downwards.

3. When returning your foot to the starting position, make sure to leave tension in the band (don't come low enough with your leg that the band becomes loose).

4. Repeat the movement while making sure your foot stays pointed downwards.

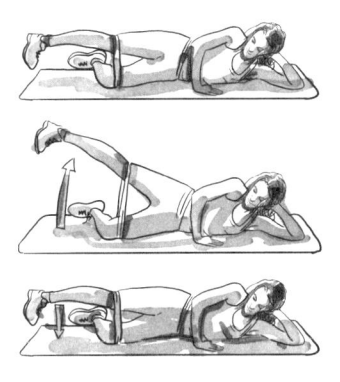

Lateral Lunge

1. Stand with your feet together.

2. Step out on one side into a lateral lunge, keeping your other foot straight.

3. Drop your butt as low as you can as if you're sitting in a chair, making sure your knees don't go past your toes in front of you.

4. From here, step back to center.

5. Repeat for duration of the set.

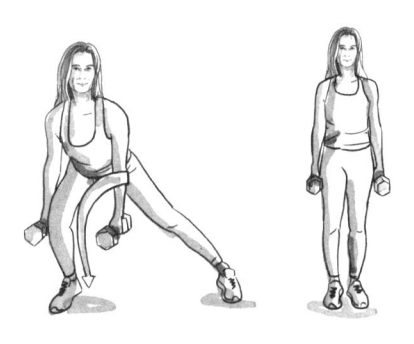

Glute Activation Warmups

Running Man

1. Wrap the resistance band around your calves or ankles.

2. Get into an athletic position with your feet shoulder-width apart, knees slightly bent and your hips dropped.

3. Move your right foot backwards while staying slightly bent, and bring it back to the original position.

4. Repeat this quickly, but feel the glute contraction every time you complete the movement.

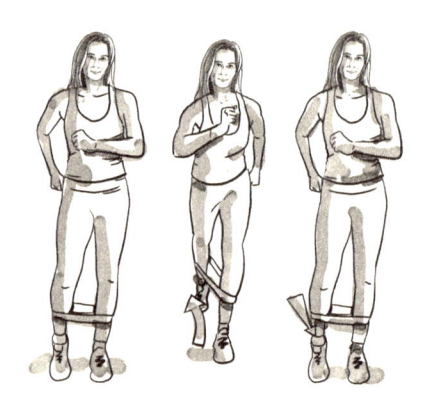

Glute Activation Warmups

Tabletop w/ Diagonal Kick

1. Get into a tabletop position with your hands and knees on the floor, and your back comfortably straight.

2. Raise one leg and straighten it.

3. As you straighten the leg, in one motion, move your straight leg behind the butt cheek on the other leg (the leg that is still on the floor).

4. Return to the original position and repeat.

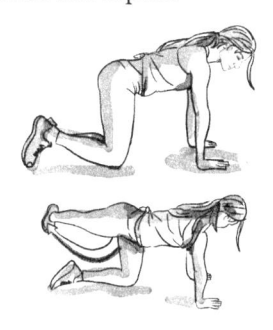

Tabletop w/ Donkey Kick

1. Get into a tabletop position with your hands and knees on the floor and your back comfortably straight.

2. Raise one leg and straighten it out directly behind you while raising it as high as you possibly can. Make sure to feel the contraction in your glute muscles.

3. Allow the leg to slowly return to the original position and repeat.

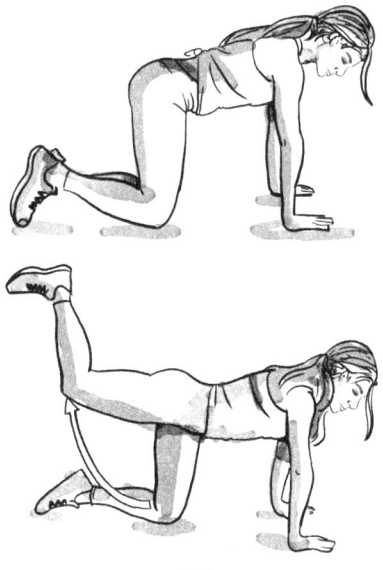

4-3-2-1 Workouts

180 Jump Twist to Floor Tap

1. Get into a squat position, and then jump up and turn 180 degrees in the opposite direction.

2. As you land on the opposite side, touch the floor all in one motion with your right arm.

3. Jump back in the other direction and touch the floor with your left arm.

4. Repeat the movement until the set is complete.

Note: You can swing your arms to propel yourself back and forth.

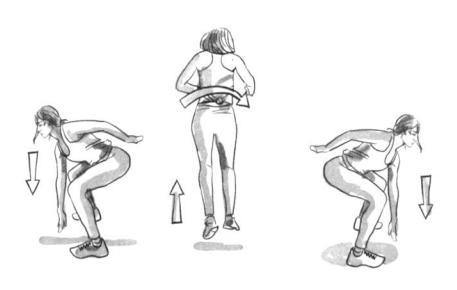

3-Point Lunge

1. Starting with your feet together and your abs pulled in, step into a lateral lunge, making sure your stabilizing foot is straight. Step back to center.

2. Using the same leg, do a reverse lunge, and then step back to center.

3. With the same leg, do a curtsy lunge, and then repeat the entire movement.

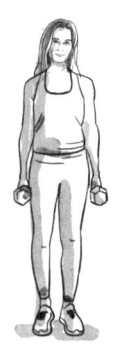

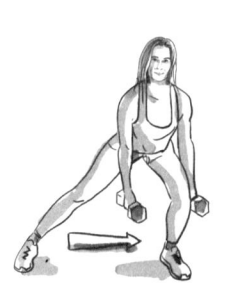

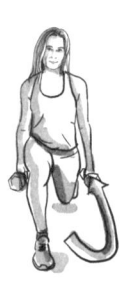

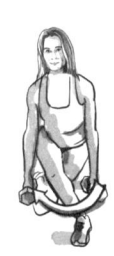

4-3-2-1 Workouts

Bulgarian Lunge

1. Place one foot behind you on a platform.

2. While your foot is on the platform, bend your other foot into a 90% lunge.

3. Push up from the lunge by driving through your front heel to return to the original position.

4. Repeat.

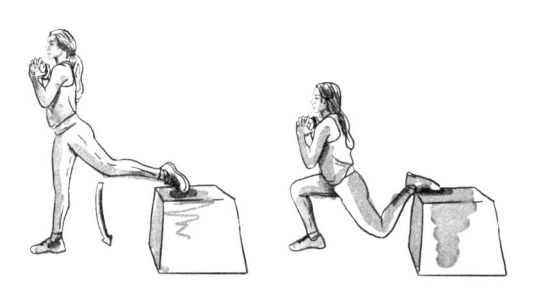

Boxing Jab

1. Standing with the knees slightly bent, hold a light dumbbell in each hand.

2. Pivot your feet to one side and jab.

3. Come back to center, and then pivot your feet to the other side and jab with your other hand.

4. Repeat the movement while continuously alternating.

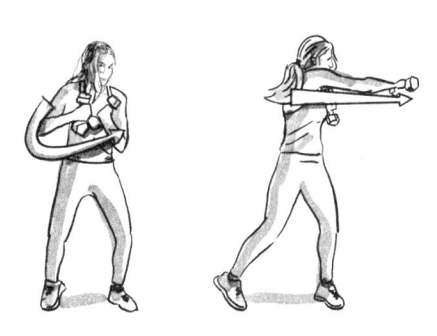

4-3-2-1 Workouts

Fast Feet

1. Start with your feet shoulder-width apart and your knees slightly bent.

2. Push through the balls of your feet and run in place, switching your feet as quickly as possible.

3. Stay low throughout the movement and move your arms as you do the running motion. Keep your spine neutral and your core tight!

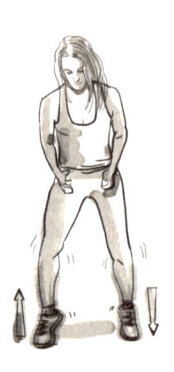

The Heisman

1. Jump or step onto your right foot and pull your left knee up towards your right shoulder as you jump.

2. Then jump onto your left foot while bringing your right knee up towards your left shoulder.

3. Repeat the movement until the set is complete.

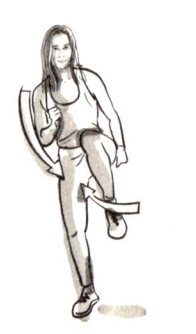

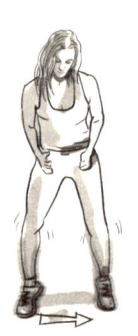

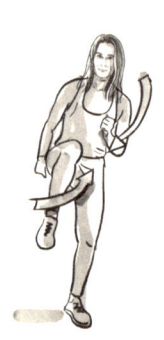

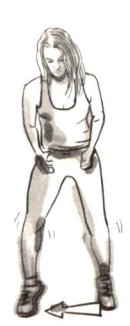

4-3-2-1 Workouts

High Knee

1. Stand straight up with your feet shoulder-width apart.

2. Run in place while raising your knees as high as possible as you alternate legs.

3. Repeat until the set is complete.

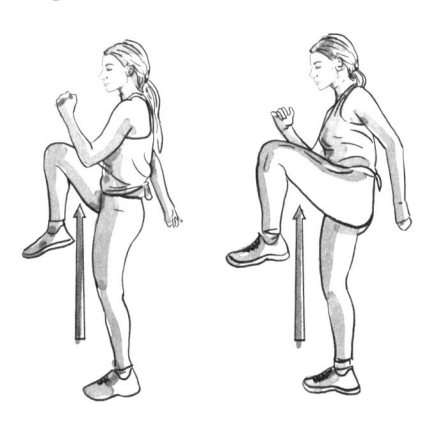

In and Out Jack

1. Stand straight up with your feet shoulder-width apart and holding dumbbells.

2. Jump into a wide squat position and touch the floor (or close to the floor) with one arm extended towards the floor.

3. Jump your feet back together in a straight, standing position.

4. Jump immediately back into a wide squat position and touch the floor with opposite hand.

5. Keep alternating arms back and forth.

*Try to keep your chest lifted while you do this.

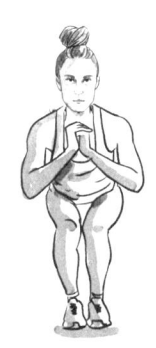

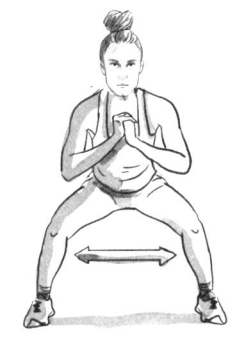

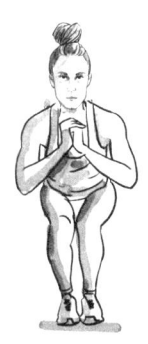

4-3-2-1 Workouts

Jump Lunge

1. Step forward into a lunge position.

2. From here, explode out of your lunge into a jump, straightening both legs.

3. As you land, lower yourself back into another lunge with your other foot in front.

4. Stay low the entire time!

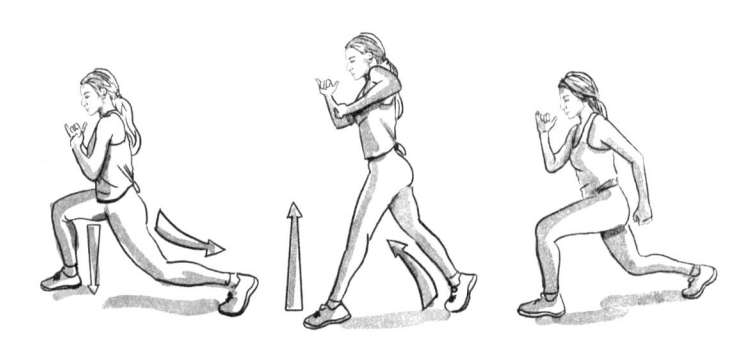

Jump Squat

1. In a squat position with feet shoulder-width apart and your weight in your heels, jump off the floor.

2. Jump then land directly back in the squat position.

3. Repeat the movement until the set is complete.

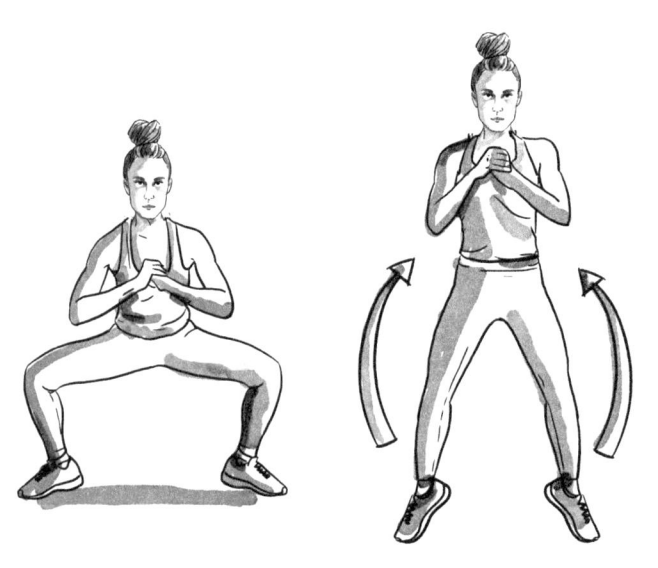

4-3-2-1 Workouts

Jump Twist

1. With your feet together, jump from side to side, while twisting your lower body.

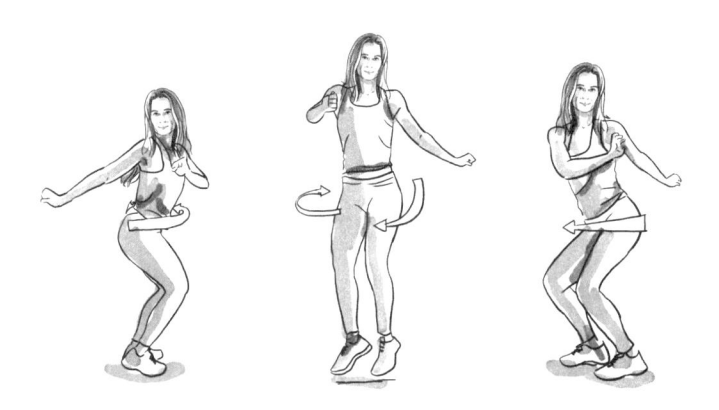

Lateral Lunge to Curtsy Lunge

1. Stand with your feet together, step out on one side into a lateral lunge, keeping your other foot straight. Drop your butt as low as you can as if you're sitting in a chair, making sure your knees don't go past your toes in front of you.

2. From here, step back to center, and with the same leg do a curtsy lunge take a big step back crossing it behind the stabilizer foot. Make sure to get your knee as close to the floor as possible!

3. Repeat for the duration of the set, and then switch sides.

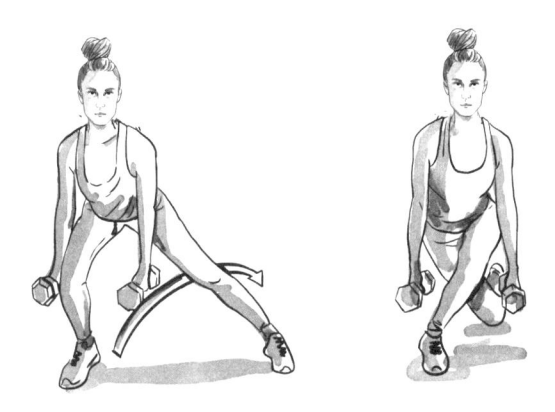

4-3-2-1 Workouts

Leg Drop

1. Lie straight on the floor or on a flat bench. Place your hands underneath your lower back or butt and push your back into the floor.

2. Raise your legs together towards the ceiling, and then slowly lower them down so that they're hovering right above the floor.

3. Bring your legs right back up.

5. Repeat.

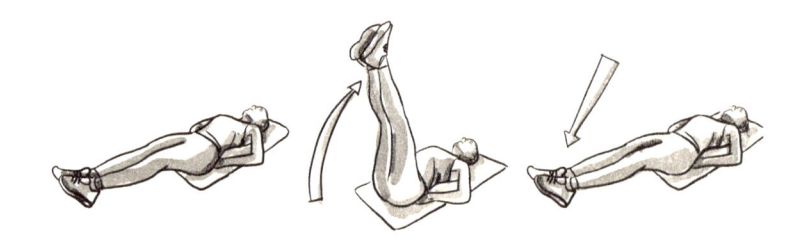

Lateral Lunge to Reverse Lunge

1. Stand with your feet together, step out on one side into a lateral lunge, keeping your other foot straight.

2. Drop your butt as low as you can as if you're sitting in a chair, making sure your knees don't go past your toes in front of you.

3. From here, step back to center, and with the same leg do a reverse lunge by taking a big step behind you. Make sure to get your knee as close to the floor as possible!

4. Repeat for the duration of the set, and then switch sides.

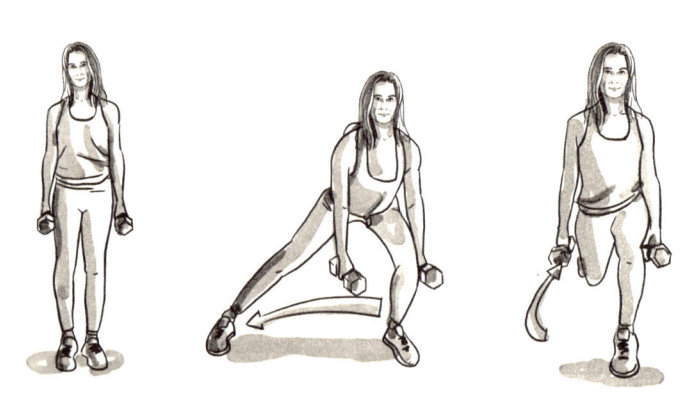

4-3-2-1 Workouts

Lateral Lunge w/ Half 'X'

1. Place a dumbbell in your left hand and step out into a lateral lunge with your right leg.

2. Next, push out of your lunge by kicking off your right leg out and extending your left arm towards the ceiling.

3. Return to the starting position and repeat.

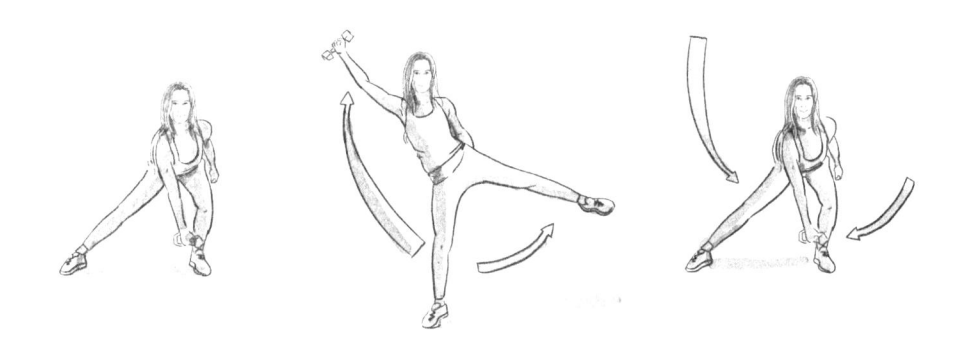

Leap Forward in Squat, Burpee, & Shuffle Back

1. Get in a squat position with your feet shoulder width apart and your hips dropped towards the floor.

2. Leap forward as far as possible while staying low in squat position.

3. Quickly put your hands on the floor.

4. Extend your feet out behind you.

5. Pop your feet back in and stand up into your squat position.

6. Shuffle your feet back in very small steps, and repeat the movement.

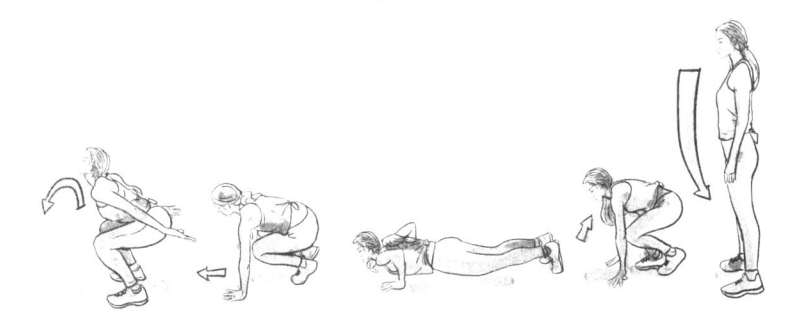

4-3-2-1 Workouts

Leg Drop

1. Lie straight on the floor or on a flat bench. Place your hands underneath your lower back or butt and push your back into the floor.

2. Raise your legs together towards the ceiling, and then slowly lower them down so that they're hovering right above the floor.

3. Bring your legs right back up.

5. Repeat.

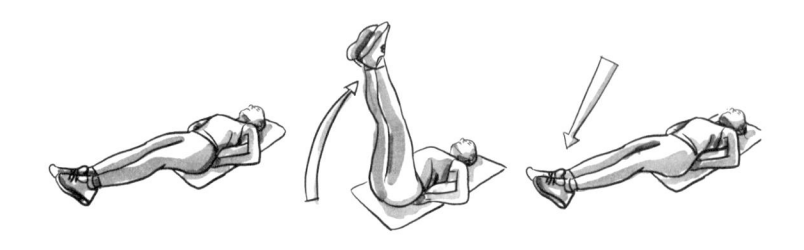

Mountain Climber

1. Get in a push-up position with your hands directly underneath your shoulders.

2. From here, jump or step your right foot as close to your right hand as possible.

3. Then immediately jump or step your left foot as close to your left hand as possible while shifting your right leg back.

4. Keep alternating your legs as fast as you can.

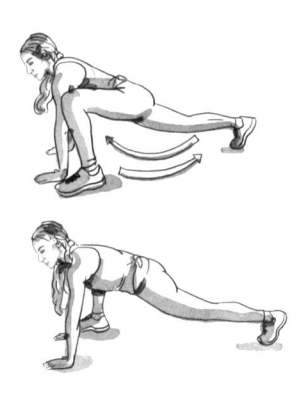

4-3-2-1 Workouts

Pendulum Jack

1. Hinge forward from your waist and place your hands on the floor in front of you.

2. Extend your right leg straight out to the side. Your left, supporting leg can be slightly bent.

3. From this position, quickly transfer your body-weight to the other leg.

4. Repeat the movement back and forth while keeping your hands on the ground until the set is complete.

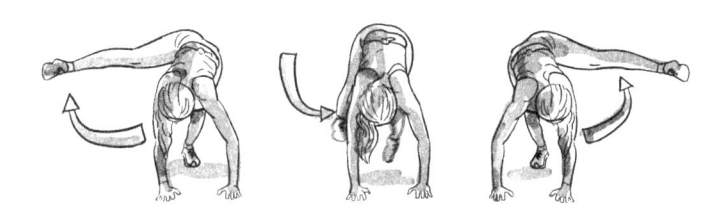

Pendulum Lunge

1. Take a large step forward until your leg is making a 90-degree angle.

2. Take the same foot that lunged forward and do a reverse-lunge.

*To challenge your balance, try keeping your leg lifted from the front lunge to the reverse lunge rather than stepping back to center.

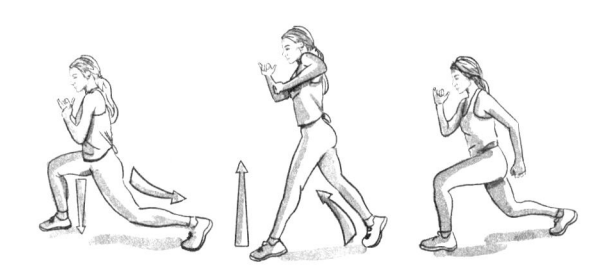

4-3-2-1 Workouts

Plank Jack

1. Get in a plank position with your hands on the floor, arms shoulder with apart and your body in a straight line.

2. From this position, jump your feet out and back in, as if you're doing a jumping jack.

*Bonus: Plank on your elbows instead of your hands to increase the difficulty of the exercise.

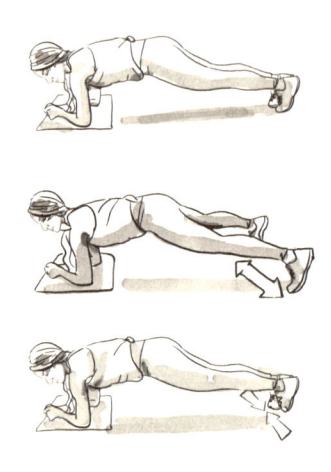

Plank Knee Tuck

1. Get in a plank position with your hands on the floor, arms shoulder with apart and your body in a straight line.

2. From this position, bring your knee from your right leg under your body and over to your left elbow.

3. Return to plank position.

4. Alternate legs and repeat for the duration of the set.

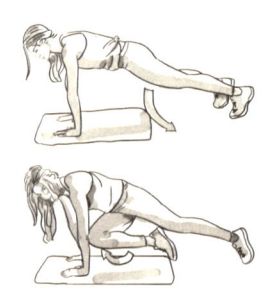

4-3-2-1 Workouts

Plank Step Up, Alternating Arms

1. Get in push-up position, but rather than have your hands on the floor, put your elbows on the floor. Keep your body straight from your head to your feet.

2. Push off your right elbow onto your hand,

3. Then push off your left elbow onto your hand so now both of your hands are on the floor.

4. Then drop from your right hand back onto your right elbow, and drop from your left hand to your left elbow.

5. Repeat the movement, starting with the left hand this time, until the set is complete.

*Keep your core tight throughout the exercise (and on all plank and leg exercises)!

*If this is difficult for you, keep your knees on the floor rather than your feet throughout the exercise.

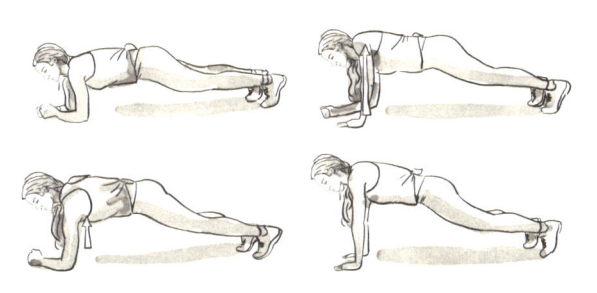

Plie Jump Squat

1. Point your toes outward so that they're facing the corners of the room, and then drop your hips into a Pile Squat position.

2. From here, jump up and then gently land directly back into the Pile Squat position.

3. Make sure your abs are pulled into your spine and your chest is lifted throughout the entire movement.

*Bonus: Touch your heels together when you are in the air.

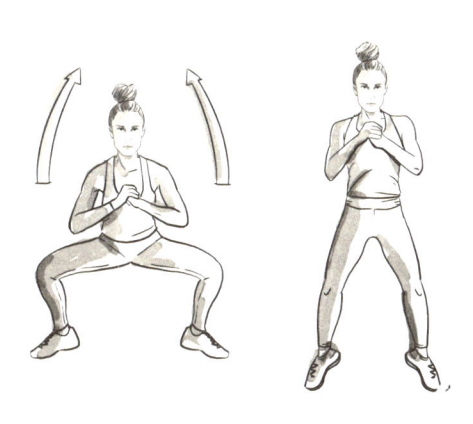

4-3-2-1 Workouts

Roundhouse Kick to Squat

1. Get into squat position.

2. Stand straight up. As you do, shift your body to the right, raise your left foot, and kick out to the left.

3. As you're bringing your leg back to the floor, enter into the original squat position.

4. Repeat until the set is complete.

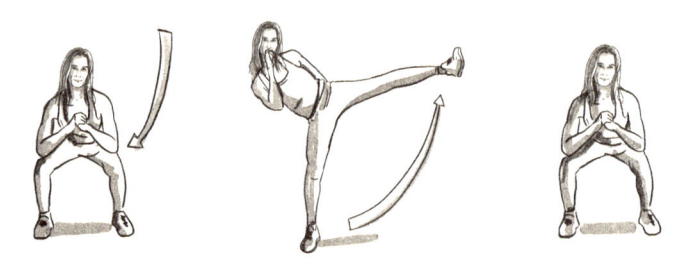

Russian Twist

1. Bend your knees and place your feet on the floor to make an imaginary 'V' shape with your body while holding yourself up. Lean your body back at a 45% angle and hold a dumbbell on both ends.

2. From here, rotate your body to one side and then shift to the other by twisting your torso.

You are never sitting straight up, you stay in the 45% angle and use your core to keep yourself stable.

Bonus: Keep your feet off the floor as you do this to work your lower abdominal muscles even more.

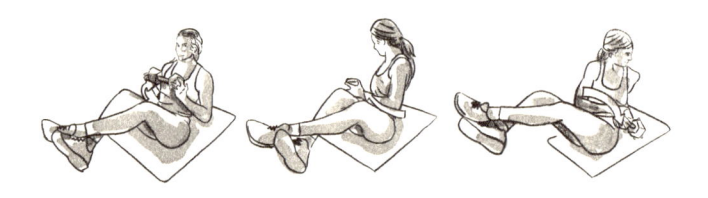

4-3-2-1 Workouts

Side Shuffle w/ Floor Tap

1. Starting in squat position, shuffle to the right three times and tap the floor.

2. Still staying low, shuffle three times to the left and tap the floor.

*Remember, stay in a low squat position throughout the whole set!

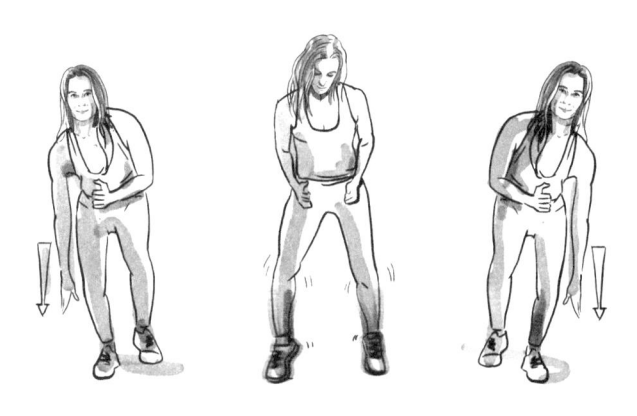

Side to Side Squat

1. Stand straight with your feet together, holding dumbbells in each hand over your shoulder.

2. Take a step out to the right, press your hips back and squat with your weight in your heels.

3. Step your feet back together, and then squat to the left.

Bonus: Hold a weight with both hands for added resistance.

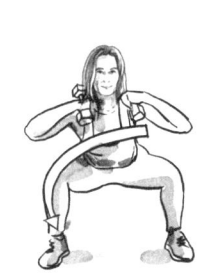

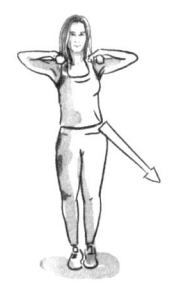

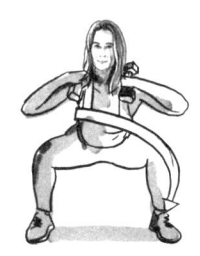

4-3-2-1 Workouts

Ski Mogul

1. Get into plank position with your feet together and jump both feet towards your right hand.

2. Then quickly jump your feet back to center position, and then jump your feet towards your left hand before jumping back to center position.

3. Keep repeating the alternating jumps until the set is complete.

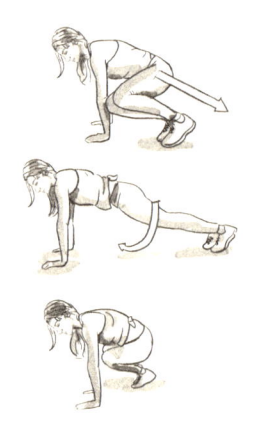

Speed Skater

1. Lean forward, jump to the right while bringing your left foot diagonally behind you, and your left arm in front of you.

2. Jump left, bringing your right arm in front of you and your right foot diagonally behind you.

3. Repeat this movement from side to side until the set is complete.

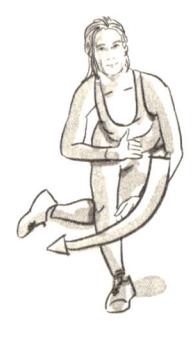

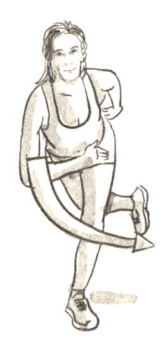

Spider-Man Plank Crunch

1. Get in plank position by placing your elbows and toes on the floor. Hold your body up off the floor in this position.

2. Bring your right knee on the outside of your body to your right elbow.

3. Straighten your right leg back to the floor.

4. Complete the same movement with your left leg and keep alternating sides.

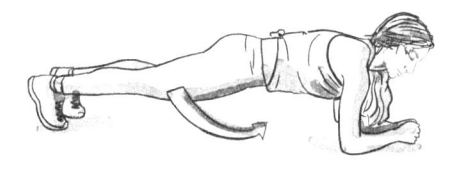

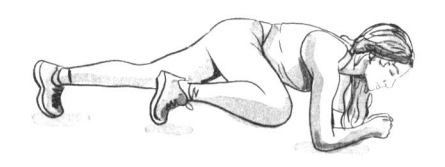

Standing Side Crunch

1. Stand with your feet a little more than hip-distance apart.

2. With a dumbbell in each hand, raise one dumbbell up and over your head - your arm should be straight.

3. From here, crunch to the side by lowering your arm while raising your knee so that your elbow and knee meet in the middle of your body. Bring your knee as far up to the side of your body as possible.

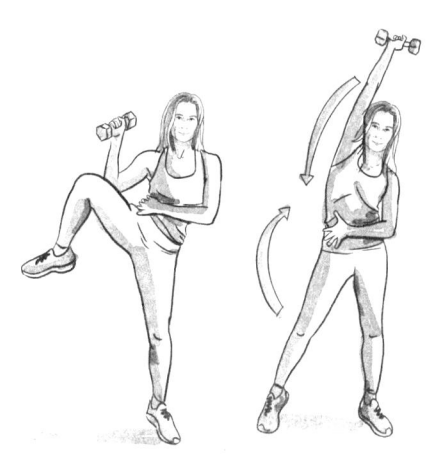

4-3-2-1 Workouts

Squat Jack

1. Stand in a squat position with your feet shoulder-width apart, knees bent and hips back towards the floor. Make sure your knees don't pass your toes.

2. From this position, jump and open your legs outwards for a bigger squat position, while staying low. Don't stand straight up in between.

3. Repeat until the set is complete.

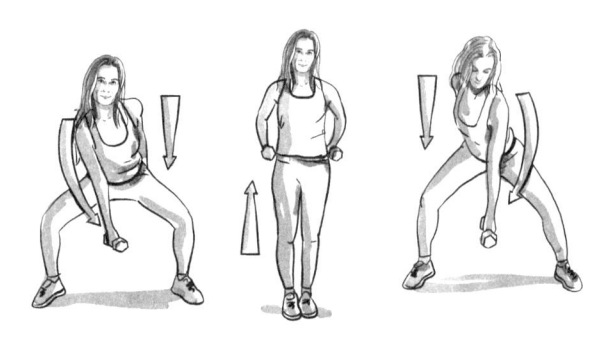

Squat Thrust

1. Stand straight up.

2. Bring both hands towards the floor, and once they're on the floor, extend both legs so they're straight behind you.

3. Jump or step your feet back to your hands.

4. Stand straight up.

5. Repeat until the set is complete!

Very similar to a burpee, just doesn't have the jump at the top.

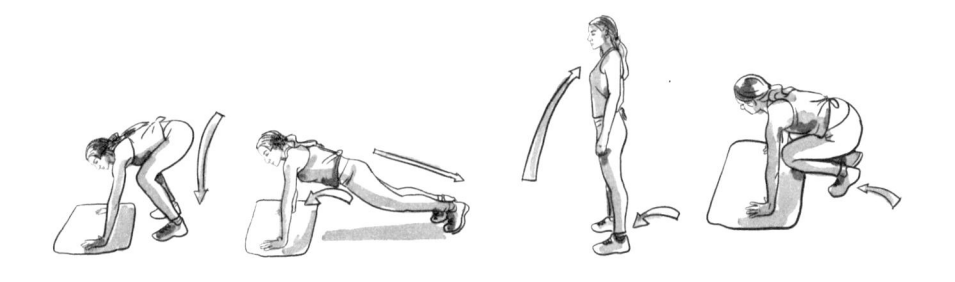

4-3-2-1 Workouts

Squat to Overhead Press

1. Holding a dumbbell on each shoulder, squat with your weight in your heels and knees aligned with your toes.

2. As you come back to starting standing position, press your dumbbells into the ceiling.

3. Return the weights to your shoulder and repeat the movement.

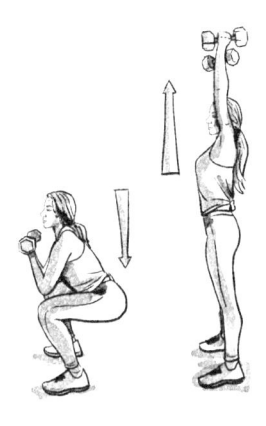

Starfish Crunch

1. Lie flat on the floor (on your backside).

2. Open your arms and legs wide to make a starfish shape.

3. Bring your left leg straight up and simultaneously bring your right hand to meet your left leg in the middle of your body, for a complete body crunch.

4. Alternate sides.

5. Repeat until the set is complete!

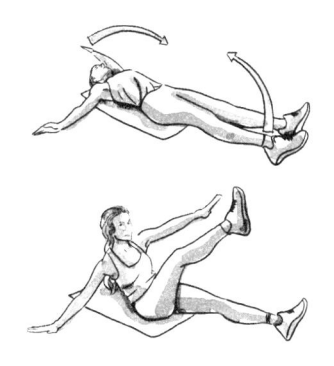

4-3-2-1 Workouts

Tabletop w/ Elbow to Knee Crunch

1. Get in a tabletop position with your hands directly beneath your shoulders. Hold your body up off the floor in this position. Hold a light dumbbell in your right hand.

2. From this position, extend your right arm out in front of you, and extend your left leg straight out behind you.

3. Next, crunch your abs by bringing your right elbow to meet your left knee in the middle of your body.

4. Extend them again and repeat.

5. Make sure to finish one side before switching hands and doing the other side.

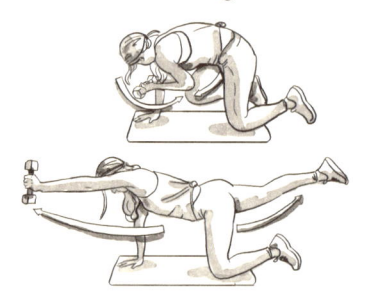

Vertical Sit-Up w/ Elbow to Knee Touch

1. Lie on your back with one leg bent and the other leg extended off the ground. Your fingertips should be behind your head.

2. From this position, twisting from the waist, get your right elbow to meet your left knee in the middle of your body.

3. Straighten your body.

4. Simultaneously bring your left knee in while raising and twisting your torso and right elbow into your left knee.

5. Repeat the movement.

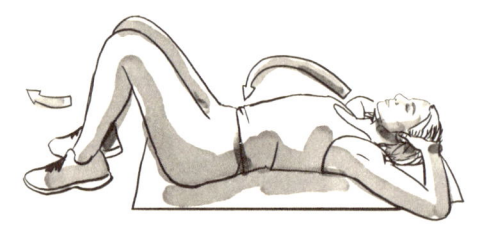

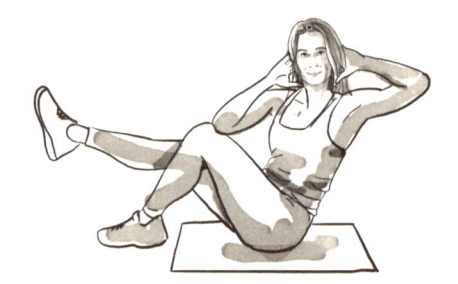

4-3-2-1 Workouts

V-Up

1. Lie straight on your back with your legs together and your arms together straight above your head.

2. In one motion, raise your legs off the floor while keeping them straight. Also raise your torso and hands to meet your legs in the middle of your body.

3. Repeat!

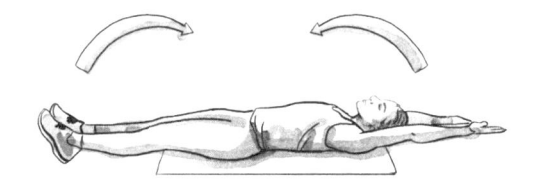

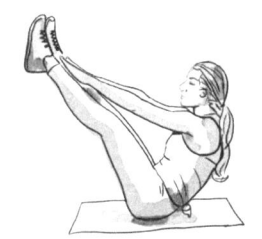

Vertical Leap

1. In a deep squat position with your weight in your heels and your booty as far back as possible, using your arms for momentum, jump up as high as you can while reaching your hands towards the ceiling.

2. Repeat this movement until the set is complete.

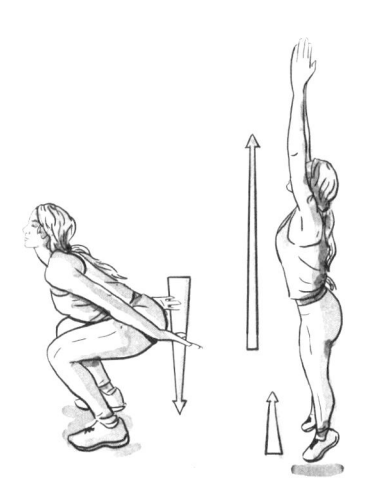

Resistance Training Exercises

Alternating Step Up

1. Hold a dumbbell in each hand, while keeping your core engaged and squeezing your glutes, step up onto a platform with your right foot (at a height that's comfortable for you,) step down, and then alternate sides.

2. Repeat.

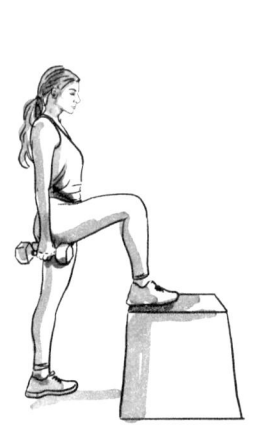

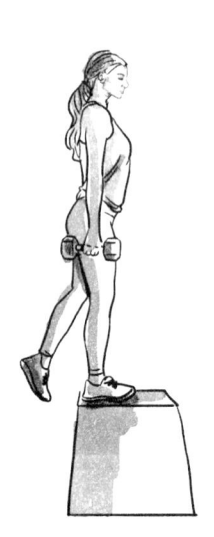

4-3-2-1 Workouts

Arnold Press

Note: This exercise can be completed sitting down on a bench or standing up. This is also combined with squats in our workouts.

1. Hold a dumbbell in each hand, raise your arms so that your palms are facing your face with your elbows close together.

3. Push the dumbbells up over your head while simultaneously twisting your hands so when your hands are straight over your head, your palms are facing outwards.

4. Bend your arms while twisting your hands so that you go back to the original position.

5. Repeat the movement!

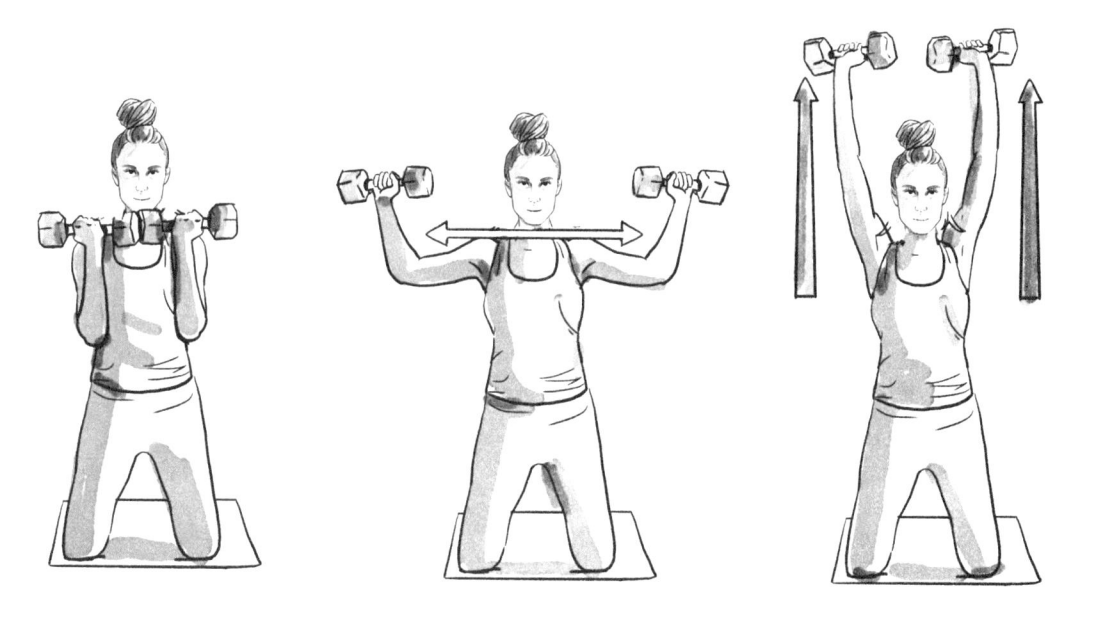

Resistance Training Exercises

Bent Over Row

Note: You can either use dumbbells or a barbell for this exercise.

1. Hold dumbbells in each hand or take a barbell and allow it to hang in front of you.
2. Hinging forward from your waist, keep your knees slightly bent and keep your back straight.
3. Drive your elbows back while squeezing your shoulder blades together. Hold for 1 second, and go back to the starting position slowly.
4. Repeat the movement.

*If you have lower back problems, try to find an alternative for this exercise like a seated row.

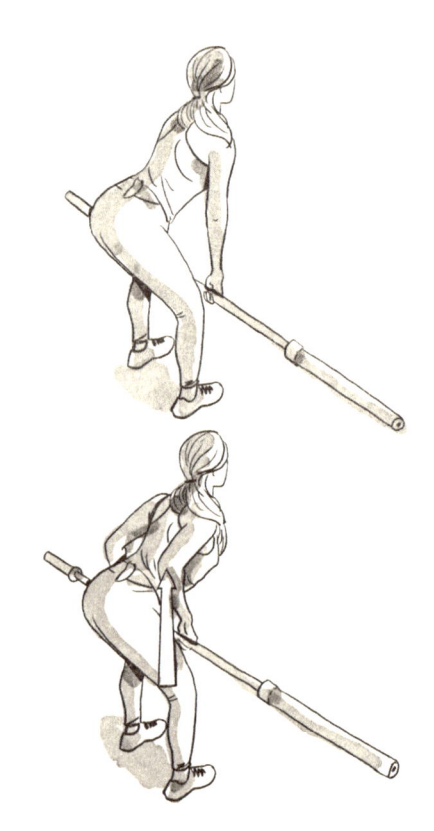

Resistance Training Exercises

Cable Row w/Squat

Caution: Avoid swinging your torso back and forth as you can cause a lower back injury.

You can use a rope, two handles, or a V-bar to complete this exercise.

1. Attach a rope to a low pulley on a cable.

2. Grab the rope and sit back in a squat position as close to 90 degrees as possible. Make sure you're far back enough that you have full range of motion with your arms.

3. Pull the rope as far back as possible by driving your elbows directly behind you. Squeeze your shoulder blades together, hold for 1 second, and then return to the starting position.

4. Repeat the movement until the set is complete.

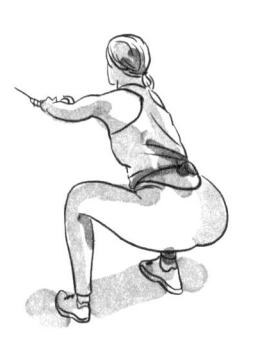

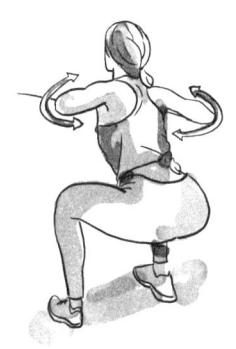

Curtsy Lunge

1. Take a big diagonal step backwards with one leg, directly crossing it behind your other (stabilizing) and lower your leg until your knee is as close to the floor as possible.

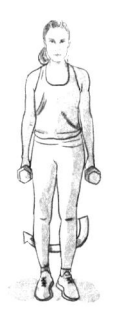

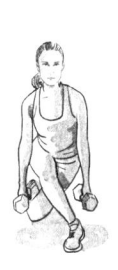

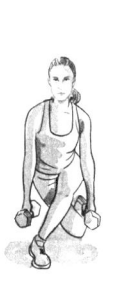

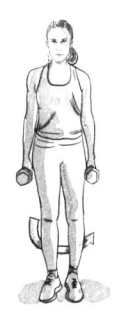

Resistance Training Exercises

Deadlift

*Note: You can do this while holding dumbbells, or with a barbell.

1. Holding dumbbells in each hand, keep your knees slightly bent and your back straight with your chest puffed outwards.

2. Hinging from your waist, bend down towards the floor as far as possible while keeping your back straight and your knees slightly bent.

3. At the climax of the movement (when you get as low as possible, hold for 0.5 - 1 second).

4. Using your legs and butt, straighten your knees until your body comes to a standing position.

5. Repeat the movement to complete the set.

*Because this exercise is more likely than others to lead to injury, please be very careful and make sure you understand proper form for deadlifts before attempting to do the exercise.

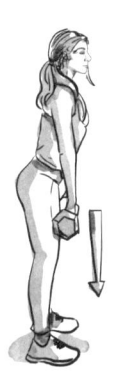

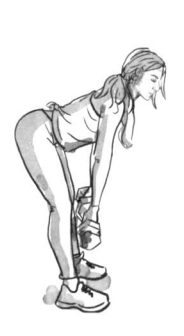

Resistance Training Exercises

Elevated Plie Squat

1. Find two platforms, boxes, or benches that you can stand on with your feet separated so that there is space in between your legs and the platforms.

2. Get into a Plie Squat position by pointing your toes outwards towards the corners of the room, drop your hips and bend your knees slightly bent.

3. Holding a heavy weight in your hands, bend your knees and drop your hips towards the floor as low as possible for a DEEP squat.

4. Slowly come back up until your knees are only slightly bent and repeat the movement.

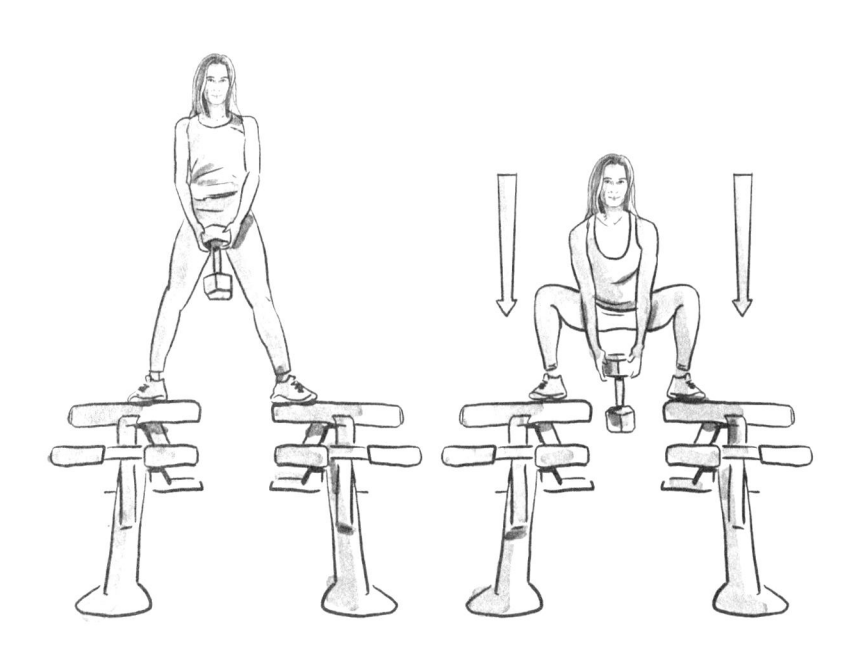

Resistance Training Exercises

Hip Thrust

1. Using a barbell or heavy dumbbell, use an amount of weight you're comfortable with.

2. Place your body under the barbell or put the dumbbell on the upper part of your thighs, and use a bench to support your back, neck, and head behind you.

3. Keep your feet on the floor, put your feet directly under your knees so that when you extend, you'll make a 90-degree angle.

4. Raise the barbell up from the floor primarily using your glute muscles.

5. Repeat the motion until the set is complete.

It is VERY important to focus on contracting your glute muscles throughout this movement - make use of the mind-muscle connection! If you need to, slightly move your feet to see if you can get your glutes to fire.

Make sure to maximize the full range of motion, going all the way up with your hips before coming back down slowly!

If you're unsure what weight you're comfortable with, start off with something very light and see how it feels. Add to it until you find that comfortable but difficult weight level.

You can use a pad or a towel under the bar for comfort

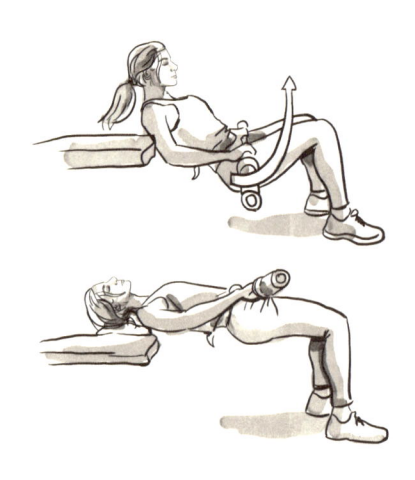

Resistance Training Exercises

Lateral Raise

*You can complete this exercise sitting down on a bench, or standing up. This is also combined with squats in our workouts.

1. Stand up straight with your feet shoulder-width apart and have dumbbells by your side at arm's-length away. When performing this exercise, your palms should be facing down.

2. Keep your abs pulled into your spine, your torso stationary, and raise the dumbbells to your side with a slight bend at your elbow. Lift your arms until they are parallel to the floor (shoulder-level) and pause for a second at the top.

3. Lower the dumbbells back down slowly and repeat.

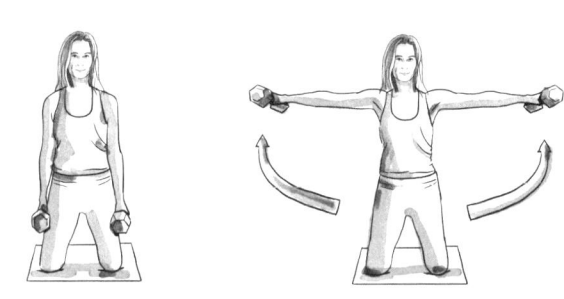

Lat Pulldown

1. Grab a wide-grip handle bar. Adjust the knee pad of the machine to fit your height to prevent your body from being raised while performing the movement.

2. Grasp the bar with an overhand grip and your palms facing forward. For a wide grip, your grip on the bar should be wider than shoulder-width apart.

3. Keep your torso stationary and pull the bar down towards your upper chest. Squeeze your back muscles during the movement.

4. Slowly raise the bar in a controlled motion back to the starting position, with your arms fully extended and lats fully stretched.

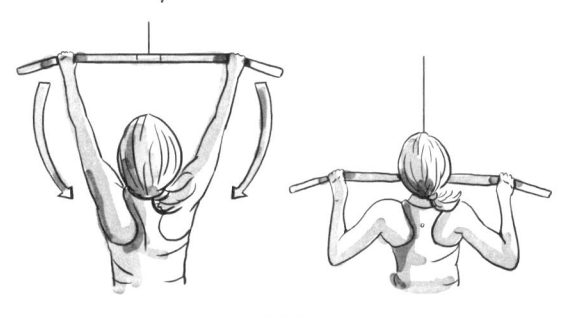

Resistance Training Exercises

Lateral Lunge w/ Knee to Elbow Rotation

1. Get into a lateral lunge position with your right leg bent close to a 90-degree angle and your left leg straight out.

2. As you push yourself out of the lunge, drive your left elbow to meet your right knee in the middle of your body. Make sure to engage your abs throughout the entire motion.

3. Repeat the movement.

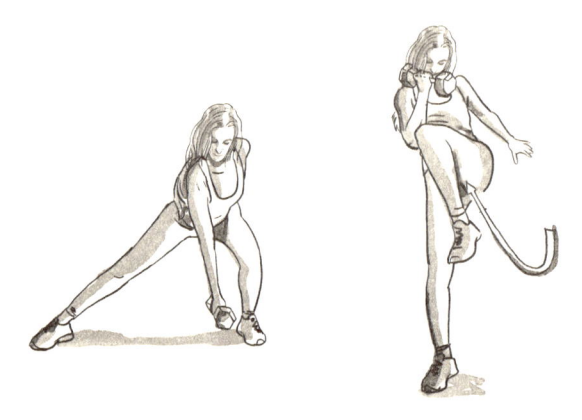

Plank to Row

1. Holding a dumbbell in each hand, get into a push-up position with your hands directly beneath your shoulders. Keep your abs pulled into your spine.

2. Drive your elbow up towards the ceiling while keeping your arm as close to your ribcage as possible.

3. Lower the weight back to the ground and complete the same movement on the other side.

4. Keep alternating until the set is complete.

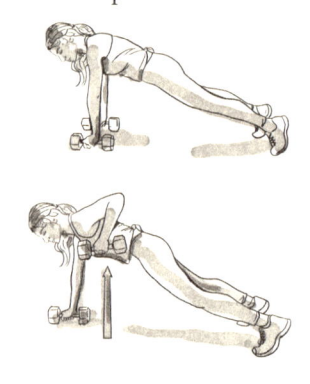

Resistance Training Exercises

Plie Squat w/ Shoulder Windmill

1. Get into a deep plie squat position with your hips dropped behind you, your knees slightly bent and feet shoulder-width apart. Feet should be pointed out towards the corners of the room.

2. Hold dumbbells in each hand with your palms facing away from your body.

3. As you squat down in this position, raise your arms up in a windmill motion, making a full circle before your hands meet over your head.

4. Staying in this deep squat, lower your arms back down in the same windmill motion, and repeat the windmill motion until the set is complete.

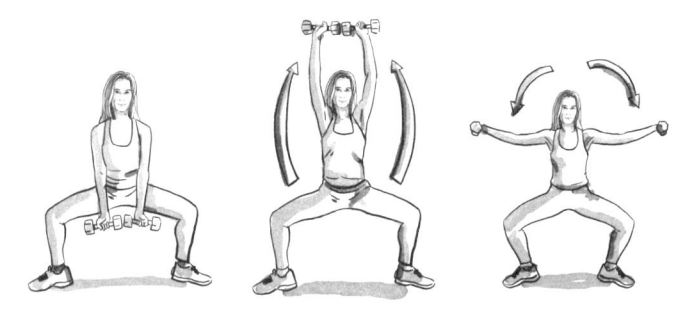

Reverse Dumbbell Fly

1. Grab a dumbbell in each hand.

2. Bend your knees slightly and hinge forward from your hips so that your upper body is leaning comfortably forward towards the floor.

3. Hold the dumbbells out together in front of your torso with your arms as straight as possible.

4. Pull the dumbbells out away from your body while keeping your arms almost fully extended, as if you were trying to squeeze your shoulder blades together.

5. Slowly return to the original position, still keeping your arms straight.

6. Repeat the movement until the set is complete!

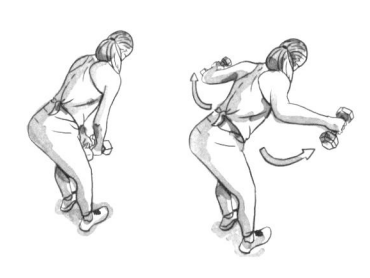

Resistance Training Exercises

Shoulder Rope Pull

1. Stand with the rope in-between your legs.

2. Keeping your arms straight (elbows *slightly* bent), pull the rope up from the floor to your shoulder height, hold for a count of two seconds, and slowly return to the starting position.

3. Repeat until the set is complete.

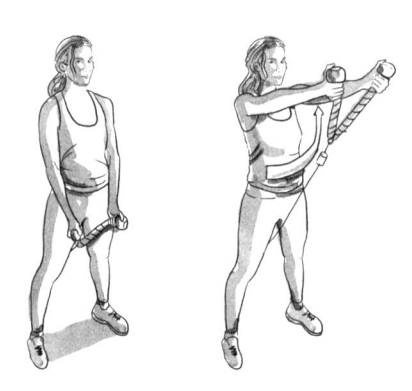

Resistance Training Exercises

Single Leg Deadlift

1. Holding dumbbells in each hand, stand on one leg, keeping the standing leg slightly bent.

2. Hinge forward from your waist so your chest is almost parallel to the floor. Use your free leg for balance by straightening outwards behind you.

3. Lift your upper body back up to the original position using your hamstrings and glutes.

4. Repeat the movement.

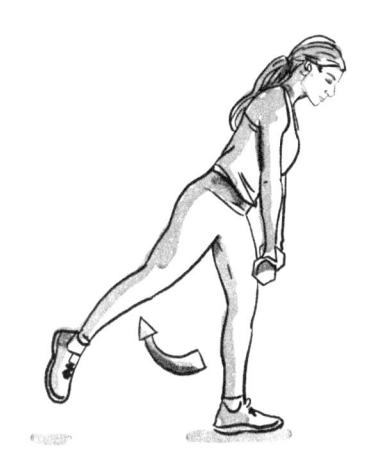

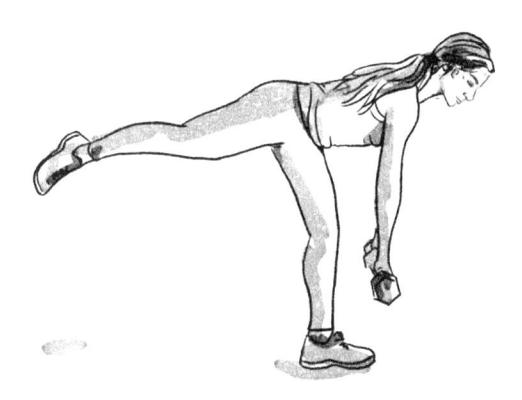

Resistance Training Exercises

Single Leg Glute Bridge

1. Lie on your back with your knees bent to a 90-degree angle. Place a heavy dumbbell on your lower stomach and hold the dumbbell on both ends.

2. Using your glute muscles, lift your hips and pelvis as high off the floor as possible.

3. With a flexed foot, straighten and lift one leg towards the ceiling - this leg stays straight in the air.

4. Lower your body down so that it almost touches the floor while keeping one leg in the air.

5. Drive your hips up as high as possible again to repeat the movement.

Make sure not to let your hips dip.

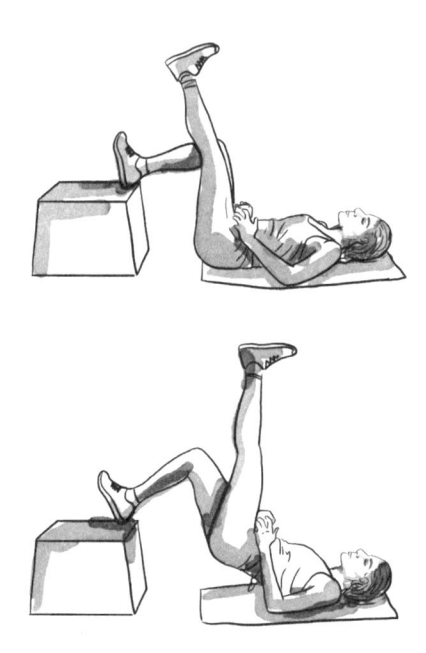

Resistance Training Exercises

Squat

1. Set a bar (barbell or Smith Machine) on the height that best works for you.

2. Step under the bar and place the back of your shoulders (just under your neck) across the bar.

3. Hold on to the bar with both arms, palms facing forward.

4. Lift up to unlock the bar by pushing your legs up and raising your torso.

5. Twist your hands back to completely unlock the bar.

6. If you're not already, stand with your feet shoulder-width apart and your knees slightly bent for a squat position.

7. Bend your knees straight down as low as possible, and step straight back up while keeping your knees in line with your heels.

If you're unsure what weight you're comfortable with, start off with something very light and see how it feels. Add to it until you find that comfortable but difficult weight level.

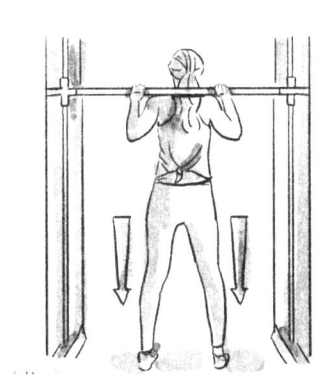

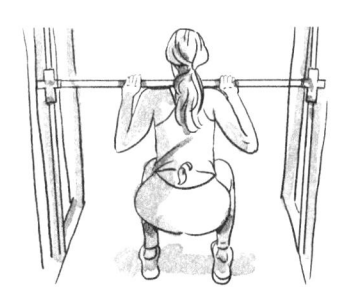

Resistance Training Exercises

Straight Arm Rope Pull or Bar Pull

The movement is the same whether you're using a rope or a bar!

1. Find a pulldown machine and attach a wide bar at shoulder-level on the pulley. Grab the bar with an overhand grip (palms facing down), and make sure your grip is wider than shoulder-width.

2. Take a couple steps back and keep your feet shoulder-width apart. Slightly hinge at the waist so your torso is leaning forward. Keep your arms fully extended, so that it's parallel with the ground, and have a slight bend at the elbows.

3. Pull the bar down while keeping the arms straight. Continue pulling down until your hands are beside your thighs; you should feel a contraction in your lats.

4. Repeat the movement.

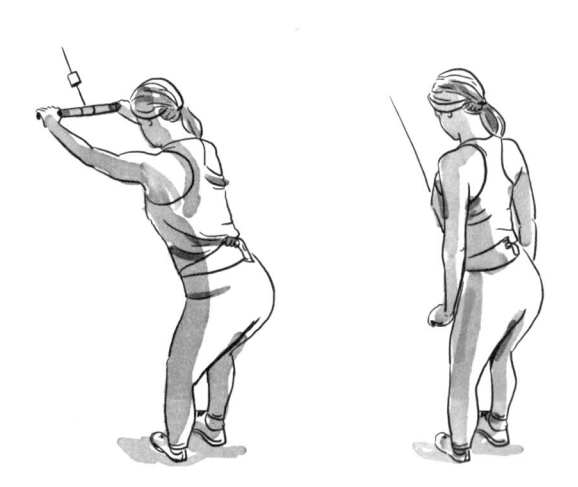

Resistance Training Exercises

Woodchopper

1. Place a dumbbell on your left shoulder, holding it with both hands.

2. Step out into a forward lunge with your right leg, bending your right knee to a 90-degree angle.

3. As you lunge, rotate the dumbbell down and across your body, making a diagonal chopping motion.

4. As you push out of the lunge and stand back up, chop the dumbbell back up to your left shoulder.

Because this exercise can sound confusing, it's worth watching a video to make sure you understand how to complete the movement!

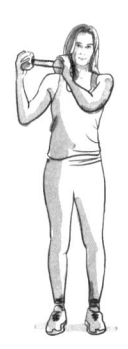

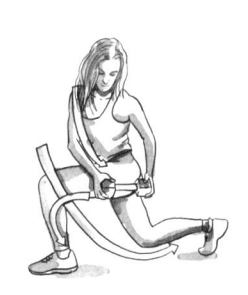

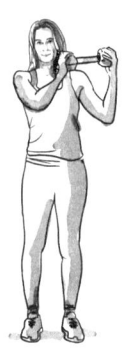

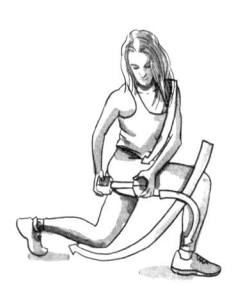

Stretches

Butterfly Stretch

1. Sit in an upright position with your back straight and your chest lifted.

2. Put the soles of your feet together and push down on your knees gently to get a deep stretch in your groin and inner thighs.

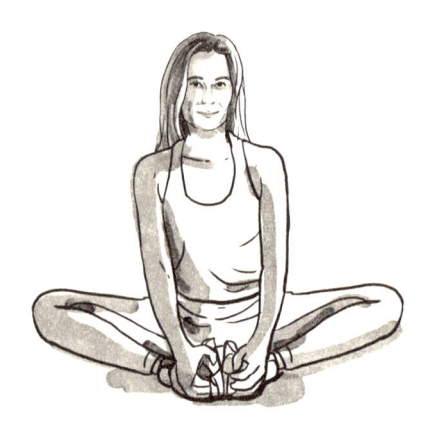

Crossbody Hangover

1. Cross one foot over the other and, hinging from your waist, hang your upper body over your lower body and try to touch the floor with your arms. Feel the stretch in your hamstrings and try to lengthen your spine.

2. Switch feet and continue the stretch.

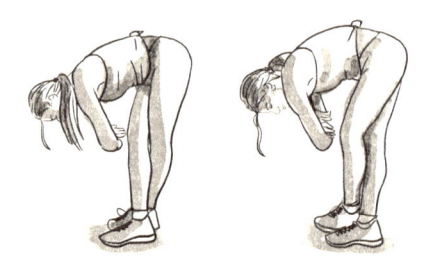

Stretches

Glute Stretch

1. Lying on your back, place one leg over the other and pull your leg towards your chest.

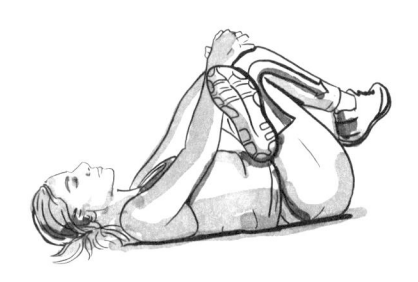

Hamstring Stretch

1. Lying on your back with one leg fully extended, bring the other leg up towards your chest while trying to keep your leg as straight as you can.

2. From here, flex and point your toes towards the ceiling. Switch legs and repeat.

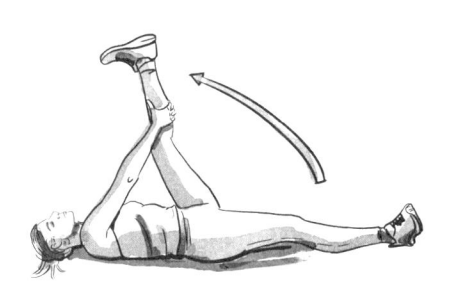

Stretches

Lat Stretch

1. Inch your fingers up the wall until you feel a stretch on the side of your body in your lats.

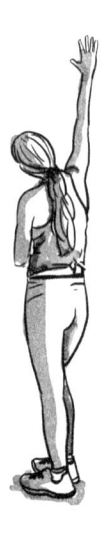

Pigeon Stretch

1. Sit with your right knee bent in front of you, and your left leg extended behind you. Pull your right heel in towards your left hip.

2. Lean forward until you feel a deep stretch in your glutes and hips.

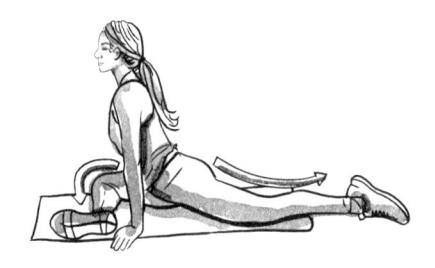

Stretches

Runner's Stretch

1. Lunge forward with one leg at a 90-degree angle while your other foot remains straight behind you with the bottom of your foot facing the ceiling.

2. Gently press through your hips. Lift your opposite arm up towards the ceiling.

3. If you're flexible enough, try lifting your foot and grabbing your toes.

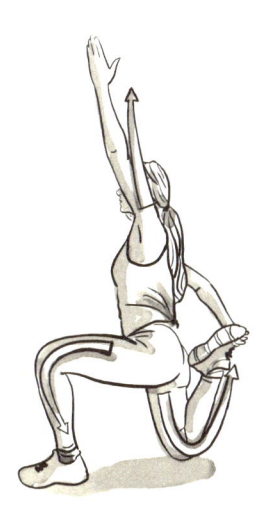